Dedication

This book is dedicated to all the people of the world who are choosing to take personal responsibility for the health and well-being of themselves and their families.

# Table of Contents

## Publisher's Note

The author and publisher have used their best efforts in preparing this book. This book is intended to provide helpful and informative material. It is not intended to diagnose, treat, cure or prevent any health problem or condition. It is not intended to replace the advice of a physician.

No action should be taken based solely upon the contents of this book. Always consult your physician or qualified health professional on any matters regarding your health and before adopting any suggestions in this book, or drawing inferences from it.

The author and publisher specifically disclaim all responsibility for any liability, loss or risk, personal or otherwise which is incurred directly or otherwise as a consequence, directly or indirectly from the use or application of any contents of this book.

Any and all product names referred to within this book are the trademark of their respective owners. None of these owners have supported, endorsed, authorized or approved this book.

Always read all information provided by the manufacturer's product manuals and labels before using their products. The author and publisher are not responsible for claims made by manufacturers.

This book is © copyrighted by Annie Deeter.

# Introduction - How We Came To Juicing

Like many people, we thought we were pretty smart about food for a good while - but the truth was, we had lost track of what was really happening with our food. We didn't know how it was produced; we knew a few things... But for the most part we were ignorant of the truth of the modern food industry. We were not suffering from any sort of critical illnesses, or grossly overweight, but we were also not bursting with energy and vitality.

We were your average couple, eating well, as far as we were concerned, but certainly not on any big health food kick, juice kick or other extreme food kick.

On my side of the equation, I'd grown up in a household where whole grains and whole foods were the norm. My mother eschewed all junk food including chips, cookies, or anything made by Hostess or any of the other name brands. We ate fruit as snack food and if we wanted cookies, we baked them. We did make a killer tollhouse chocolate chip cookie around our place - and everyone in the family could pull it off - so we were not without the experience of cookies; just not as a common daily event.

Instead, mom read Adele Davis and bought no junk food, period. Well, except for the very occasional box of Nabisco Ginger Snaps, which she indulged in for herself, and kept hidden up in a high cupboard, so we really didn't even know she did this until we were old enough (and tall enough!) to discover them. She was always completely crazy for ginger.

My husband had a similar upbringing in Europe and was unaccustomed to American junk food, so we really thought we were 'on top of it' in the food department. Oh, we let the kids have frozen pizza now and again, and we kept frozen pot pies and burritos on hand for them when they were in high-school and college and working, as a fast bite to eat - but basically, we were clueless.

We had always been a family that sat down to dinner together and had plenty to talk about as we did so. I guess we figured that this was pretty good for a culture where so many were eating fast food, not even seeing each other at meal-times and hardly ever sitting down to eat together. And we certainly kept the kitchen stocked with plenty of fresh fruits and vegetables.

But things were changing in the world, and we were just beginning to get an inkling that all was not well in the world of food.

Then our youngest son spent a year in the Culinary Arts School at his college and began to re-invent our old whole foods approach, preferring nothing so much as a whole peeled cucumber for a snack.

Our world began to change. We began shopping at the local farmers markets again, and making a lot more fresh salads.

Around this same time, we came across the work of Dr. Max Gerson, and began to read about his amazing juicing and healing protocols. We were impressed by the stories of his healing such luminaries as Albert Schweitzer; and began reading about his work and the work of his daughter Charlotte Gerson. We discovered the Gerson Institute.

Another important event radically shifted our thinking shortly thereafter. Our culinary arts student son insisted we needed to watch a new film that had just come out called "Food, Inc."; and we did.

From then on, our world began to change very rapidly in the world of food, and we have never looked back.

One of the best, most long standing and useful changes we have made to our food and eating regimen is the addition of regular juicing of fresh organic vegetables, herbs and fruits to our diet. In many ways, this one change has been more profound than any other.

First, there is absolutely no doubt that it has given us a whole new level of energy and well-being. Second, it has taught us that we have a solution when life gets hectic and high stress. Whenever we are pressed by deadlines or even just have a heavy physical schedule (moving house, for example) juicing can give us the stamina to get the job done. Not just get it done, but do so without exhausting ourselves. Juicing gives us the energy we need to stay cheerful and in control of the situation, avoiding overwhelm and the emotional strain that can occur when stress is high.

It is remarkable to think that we did without this incredible energy and health boosting opportunity for so long, actually. But no more!

No question we are enthusiastic when it comes to juicing. However, we note that many people seem to have a resistance to the idea. Perhaps it is seen as a 'fad' or some kind of 'trick' or simply 'too good to be true' and therefore not worth trying out.

It is our hope that anyone who encounters this book will at least give it a try. Adding juicing to your diet can provide you with increased energy and stamina right away, even if you don't manage to juice every day.

In the years since our adventure with juicing began, our lives have changed dramatically. We no longer shop in the chain grocery stores. We buy local and organic. We fish, and we grow a big garden. We buy local fruits and grass fed pasture raised meats raised in our own community. We are, at this point, complete foodies, totally committed to our local food shed and the

13

importance of local food security and sustainability. We've more or less revolutionized our eating and food buying and procuring ways.

Now this doesn't mean everyone who drinks fresh home-made vegetable and fruit juices will follow in our foot-steps, and we are not suggesting that - we just look back sometimes and marvel at how much our lives and our eating habits have changed in those few short years since Brad went to culinary arts class!

We consider ourselves very fortunate. Were it not for our kids and their influence and our willingness to pay attention, we might be victims of the modern food industry, which seems set on poisoning us all. But not us. We are healthy, happy, full of energy and having a great time of life. For the most part, we don't get sick, we don't get depressed and we don't have allergies or other ailments which seem to plague so many in our modern culture.

We know we are blessed and we are grateful. And in large part, we owe our biggest gratitude to Max Gerson and his daughter Charlotte, who, by their example and the Max Gerson Therapy, set us on our way to becoming avid juicers.

We are, by nature, investigators on many levels, a researcher and an engineer, we are the kind of people who love nothing more than a good detective story of the real kind. Excited by understanding how and why and what makes things work. We both get great satisfaction from discovering how to make things better. So perhaps it was only a matter of time and we would have ended up here anyway. But thanks to our health conscious youngest son and a few great books and films, we were catapulted into a new way of thinking and living around food that has served us very well and made all the difference in the quality of our lives.

This is the story of our exploration into the world of juicing, how we decided upon the Omega Juicer and what we have learned along the way. We hope it provides useful insights and helpful information for anyone considering the path of juicing, and in particular, anyone who is interested in the Omega Juicer.

Before moving on, it must be stated that we have no connection to the Omega Juicer company, any of its employees, executives, advertising staff or anything like that. Our sole connection to the company is that we are happy customers of their juicer. We are not endorsed, supported or in any way authorized by them or by anyone else to write this book. We decided it should be written because we are enthusiastic juicers and we love our Omega Juicer. That's it. No strings attached.

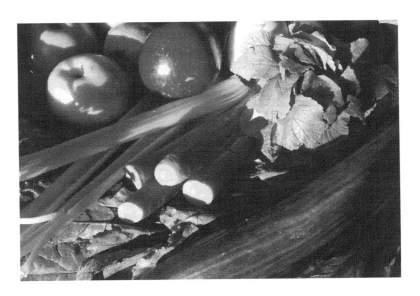

## Juicing - What It Is, What It's Not, and Why That Matters

Plenty of people have heard of juicing by now, and plenty more have a complete misunderstanding of what it is.

This is due in part to chain stores like Jamba Juice, who, while they do offer a limited number of actual vegetable juices, namely sell ice-based fruit smoothies. These smoothies are made of various frozen and fresh food products blended in a high-speed blender. Whenever you take whole fruits, vegetables or any parts thereof, and throw them into a blender and whip them up into a frothy concoction, you are making a smoothie. This might seem like nit picking but really it is not.

Smoothies contain the whole kit and caboodle of whatever the ingredients are that go into them. Naturally, you peel the oranges or citrus, just as you do in juicing, but the difference is that the end result contains all the parts of the fruit or vegetable, just all blended up. There is absolutely nothing wrong with this, honestly.

It's just not juicing.

The Omega Juicer allows you to do real juicing. In real classical juicing, aka Max Gerson style, or the real nutritionist style of juicing, the fiber is separated from the liquid of the fruit or vegetable during the juicing process. The fiber is extruded separately and is very dry, while the liquid is extracted and drained off into the juice-receiving bowl or cup.

The reason this is an important distinction is that when the nutritional components are separated from the fiber, the juice that is produced is extremely nutrient dense and instantly bio-available. What this means is that as the juice enters your mouth, the cells of your tongue and surfaces inside your mouth can literally take in those nutrients instantly. Furthermore, nutrients will be delivered to specific parts of your digestive system exactly as appropriately needed. In some cases, this means nutrients will retain their complexity throughout the early digestive processes in order to deliver specific functionality to the large intestine.

You can actually feel this difference when you drink a juicer-created juice. It hits your palate and instantly the nutrients are flowing into your blood stream from every surface it comes in contact with as it moves through your body. In fact, when you first begin juicing, you may discover that this action is so fast that your digestive system is stimulated almost immediately upon drinking your juice. But don't let that dissuade you, or cause alarm. It's natural. Your body's entire system is stimulated and put into action as you begin to drink the juice.

In the beginning, this can cause concern for some people, who might suppose something is wrong with them, or with the idea of juicing. This is not so. It is simply your body's reaction to a super nutrient dense and extremely bio-available food. Taking your time to sip the juice slowly, starting with smaller servings and continuing to juice regularly, will all work to reduce the 'instant' response. The good news is, this is your body's way of telling you that the juice is working. Your body is responding quickly to a powerhouse of nutritious and healing food extracts. This is what it really is, after all, when you extract the nutrients in their liquid form from the various fruits and vegetables.

You can think of it this way: it's a sign that the juice is working and your body is responding appropriately. Depending how far from such direct nutrient intense experiences your body has strayed, your experience will be more or less intense.

Over time, this instant digestive response will diminish, although juicing will do wonders for anyone with a sluggish bowel.

Once you become a regular juicer, your digestion will level out and you'll be less prone to such an 'instant' response. You will stay regular and find you have fewer issues with constipation or diarrhea as well.

There are those who caution that juicing is dangerous because you are eliminating the fiber and therefore somehow creating a problem for your body. This is simply not true. First off, you are not only consuming juice as a complete diet, unless you are doing a short term fasting program, and second, there is nothing intrinsically harmful about giving your body super nutrient-packed vegetable and fruit juices extracted from whole organic foods.

Just realize that the benefits of real juicing come from separating and releasing the nutrients from the cells of the fruits and vegetables, and not blending them together. For those looking to increase fiber in their diet, the fiber extracted when juicing can be used in soup stocks and stews to increase fiber content, or frozen for later use. The fiber can also be composted, added to the garden, or fed to poultry and/or pigs.

This brings us to the next issue with juicing which is all about juicer types and how different juicers work. This, in fact, is what led us to the Omega Juicer in the first place.

# Different Types of Juicers - Masticating and Centrifugal

There are essentially two different approaches to extracting juice from fruits, vegetables, grasses, herbs and/or roots. Although they both result in juice separated from the fiber of the item being juiced, they accomplish it in completely different ways.

The first is the masticating juicer. This type of juicer uses a slow rpm (revolutions per minute) and either a single or double gear system which uses pressure to quite literally 'chew' or squeeze and crush the juice out of whatever is being juiced. Many of these juicers can also be used to make nut butters, baby foods and even frozen desserts.

The second type of juicer is a centrifugal juicer. This type of juicer first breaks up the item to be juiced into small pieces and then extracts the juice through a high speed centrifugal action which spins the juice out of the fiber pieces.

The principles of their actions are completely different: one is moving very slowly to crush the juice out of the fruit or vegetable; one is breaking the fruit or vegetable up and then spinning out the juice.

The major differences which really matter between these two approaches are: one is low heat, and slow pressure. The other uses fast spinning which introduces heat. The result is that the slower and heatless process produces more juice from each thing juiced and can also juice grasses and fine leaves. The centrifugal juicer is not effective at juicing grasses or fine leaves (barley grass, wheat grass, parsley, mint, spinach etc.). Because it relies on a high speed spinning action, these more delicate plant structures are not completely juiced and the pulp or fiber extruded has a much higher liquid content, meaning the juice is being left in the fiber and not fully extracted. It also, through its spinning action, introduces a lot more oxygen into the juice; as well as heat. The oxygen causes the juice to oxidize, or break down, much faster. The heat introduced in the high speed spinning destroys some of the nutritive value of the juice.

Both forms of juicing will work. However, for the best nutrition content of the resulting juice, a masticating juicer is preferable. Without heat, it can retain the highest living content of the enzymes, vitamins and nutrients in the juice. Its slow action does not incorporate oxygen into the juice leaving the juice able to be stored for up to a few days without degradation.

When oxygen is introduced to the juice, the vital nutrients begin to break down immediately, and the juice must be consumed right away and cannot be stored for later use.

## How we chose the Omega Juicer

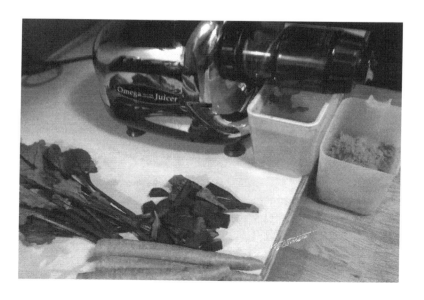

For all of these reasons, and based on our research at the time, including the Gerson Therapy recommendations and others, we determined that the best juicer for our money would have to be a masticating juicer. While they are more expensive, they are also more durable and longer lasting, having no high rpm moving parts. We settled on a single gear masticating juicer as the best choice for our needs based on the factors of durability, ease of use and highest nutritive value of juice.

Finally, because the masticating juicer does not incorporate oxygen into the juice, we would be able to make juices and store them in the refrigerator for up to three days, eliminating the need for daily juicing without giving up the opportunity to have fresh juices every day to drink.

# Getting Started with Juicing - A few things we got right

Most Americans have developed a palate which is shaped by sweet and salty. This is not because we are bad cooks or even because we are naturally self-indulgent. It is a direct result of the industrial food which inundates our shops and selection choices.

Anyone who understands that McDonald's hamburgers have sugar in them has an idea of how this works, and can begin to appreciate that our palates are being shaped based on the desires of an industry which desires to sell us particular foods or food-like products, as they have been called.

There is a good and a bad side to this situation. The bad is that we are conditioned to eating things which have been designed purposefully to trigger our sweet/salt cravings and to accentuate our awareness of them, so that things which are not a match to this over-exaggerated sweet/salty food design seem bland, bitter or unpleasant tasting to our palate.

The good news is that this natural tendency towards the sweet and salty ends of the taste spectrum derives out of our natural affinity for things which match this profile, and when not over exaggerated, are signals to our brain regarding the nutritive values of real foods. In other words, carrots and beets and yams are naturally very sweet when juiced and our palate responds to this natural sweetness exactly as it should - it likes it. Which is a very good thing, because all three of these foods contain vital nutrients our bodies crave.

(A quick note on yams: In the United States, "yams" are actually orange-fleshed, red-skinned sweet potatoes. The most common varieties are Jewel, Garnet, and the new Georgia Jet, a cold hardy variety which can be grown throughout the United

States. True yams are grown throughout Africa and parts of Asia where night time temperatures never go below 70°F. Sweet potatoes are much more nutritious than true yams, see the juicing ingredients guide in this book for more details.)

When it comes right down to it, our bodies and our brains crave foods which are naturally very high in nutrition and which have tastes which reflect this high nutritive value.

Just because our brains and taste buds have been tricked into eating substitutions which are full of air and void of nutrition does not mean our apparatus is defective. Indeed, quite the contrary is true.

One of the great benefits and joys of juicing is that the further down the road of juicing you go the more your brain and palate will provide you with the absolute undeniable positive feedback that they LIKE THIS STUFF and YOU SHOULD DO MORE OF IT! It is incredible how, after only a short time, you will find yourself craving these juices rather than the artificial foods and food products which have captured your palate, your brain and your pocketbook for the last several decades at least.

On the other side of this coin are the bitters. Bitter vegetables, plants, herbs, and foods hold an important and historically powerful place in our digestion and overall health. Yet, for the most part, our modern palates have been trained away from bitter. Well, unless we want to talk about coffee, that is!

But for most people, organically grown pungent celery and the bitter greens (mustards, collard, kale etc.) taste unpleasantly bitter and are not something they are rushing out to purchase and consume large quantities of, because, well... they're bitter!

However, it is precisely their bitter qualities which make these foods the cleansing, purgative, nutritionally important foods they are.

So, for most people the idea of juicing things like barley grass, celery, kale or collard greens is nothing short of unappealing. Anyone who has had a majorly strong green juice knows that there is a level of pungent 'green'-ness which goes over the top, fills your sinuses and can actually make you gag. Or, as one juicing enthusiast wrote when describing how to deal with this problem "How to make a green juice that doesn't feel like a face plant in the lawn." - Indeed.

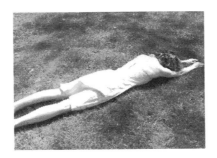

And yet, we know the greens in these green juices are what make them so healthy and vital for us.

Our advice?

When you start juicing, do not try to go to the far extremes of green juicing as your first step.

Recognize that your palate has been shaped by forces beyond your control in the short-term immediate past, and go slow. The best and easiest way we found to do this is to start with a basic juice of carrot, celery and orange or apple. 1 medium orange or 2 small apples, 4 medium carrots and 4 medium stalks of celery make a nice 12oz. drink for one person.

In the early days of our juicing we would pick up a 2lb bag of carrots, two bunches of celery and four to six apples and juice it all at once and mix it up to taste until we liked it. Generally we liked it pretty much no matter how we mixed it up, because the apple tempers the celery nicely and the carrot is sweet already.

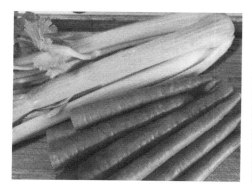 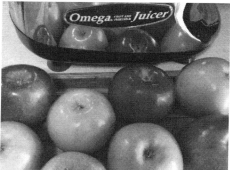

Next start adding sweet potatoes, beets and cucumbers and see what you think of that. The sweet potatoes and beets are sweet, and that gives room to add more of the kales, barley grasses and other sharp greens which balance them.

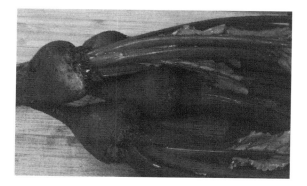

Adding orange and lemon is always a benefit and always delicious and in fact one of our favorite things to do is to add orange, lemon and lime - whewie what a zing! Plus the vitamin C will improve the body's absorption of the iron and calcium in those leafy greens.

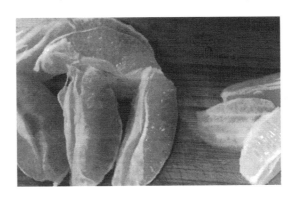

Most important of all, keep playing around as you get started. Why? Because the absolute worst thing that you can do at this early stage of juicing is to listen to some 'guru' or take some 'expert advice' which convinces you to make up juices for which your palate is not yet adapted or ready and then stop juicing altogether.

Oh, and by the way, if you are a parent, this is doubly and triply true for your kids. Start them off with yams, beets and carrots and maybe throw in a lemon or some celery (not too much!) so they get that super sweet YUMMO taste that has them BEGGING for more. You can work to help them adjust their palate later. And they will - because the real power and beauty and JOY of juicing is that the more you do it the more your palate and your brain and your body wake up and get in the picture and insist you do more of it. It's a totally natural phenomenon and it will lead you effortlessly to better health and well-being.

## Mistakes of Newbie Juicers

While it would be fun to say that we were expert juicers from the start, it would be a flat out lie.

You'd think, with all our research and planning, and given that we actually bought our Omega Juicer as a Christmas present to each other, we'd have been ready to dive in and get it right, right from the start. You'd be wrong.

It's funny, isn't it? But whenever you start something new, you seem to expect to know everything there is to know about it before you begin and you forget, or at least we do, that anything new is, well, new.

Learning a new skill or practice always starts with the first time you attempt it. Yet, we as humans seem to think we can skip that first step and just go right to 'experts' on our first go. Too funny.

Well, we were no different when it came to juicing.

We got our beautiful shiny new Omega Juicer and set right to work.

We spent hours chopping up carrots and celery and apples into nice little bits. We spent more hours carefully and tediously feeding those little bits into the machine and hoping against hope that we were not over taxing the machine with too many little bits at a time.

The thought of this still makes us laugh out loud. Really? Really! We did what all men are always accused of, no matter the culture or age, it seems. We failed to even READ the instructions! We just assumed we were experts and dove right in. Chop chop chop.

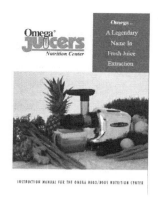

These days the idea of cutting up a carrot or anything that already fits into the feeder for the juicer is so laughable we still get a giggle out of ourselves whenever we use our juicer.

It wasn't until a couple of months went by, and my husband went home to visit his parents in Europe that we got the wakeup call and another good laugh.

Turns out, in his excitement about juicing, my husband had told his parents all about our adventures and had not left out the endless chopping on the cutting board. His father had smiled warmly, and suggested that he had just seen a television show where they were demonstrating this newfangled thing called juicing, and the people on that show were not chopping up anything unless it didn't fit into the opening for the juicer...

They were feeding whole carrots and stalks of celery right into the machine and getting juice and pulp out the other end! Imagine that.

Of course I had to try it before he even got home. And, of course, it worked just fine.

No more chopping.

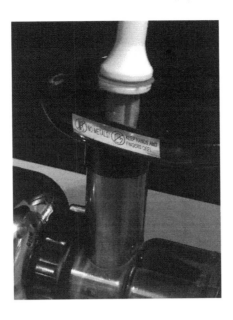

Now, what's really funny is that some months later we actually sat down and read the Omega juicer manual - and guess what? They suggest that 'to get the most out of the vegetables you juice you should cut them all up into small pieces'. Forget it. Unless you have hired help with nothing to do, or nothing to do yourself most of the time, just do not even go there. The closest we come to cutting things up is to split large carrots lengthwise, or maybe even quarter them lengthwise, but that's it. Otherwise the only chopping you do is to fruits and vegetables which are round (and therefore will not fit into the juicer without slicing them up a bit).

We've been juicing this way for a few years now and it works just fine. One thing we do pay attention to, when it comes to the manual is not to ever run the juicer for more than 30 minutes at a time without shutting it off and letting it rest. But most of our juicing sessions take a lot less than 30 minutes of continuous running of the juicer. The only time we have to watch the clock is when we are going on travel or something and are making juice to last the next two days or so (we generally do not ever store juices longer than 3 days).

All our worries that the machine would not be able to handle whole carrots or celery stalks or whatever portions of an apple would fit into the top of the chute were for naught. This machine was, after all, built to juice fruits and vegetables! There is no discernible difference in the pulp extruded from cut up vegetables or whole vegetables, that is no extra juice is left in the pulp.

So do yourself a favor, and don't waste time chopping everything up into little bits for your juicer. IF they will fit into the juicer, the juicer will juice them.

The other big mistake we made early on is related, in a strange way.

It is again, that failure to recognize a new experience and keep it open to experimentation instead of locking it into a way of doing things, or a fast and hard set of rules before you've had time to even play around a while.

We fell into a rut.  You'd have thought the only vegetables on the planet approved for juicing were carrots and celery! Who had ever heard of anything else? Oh, sure, we'd juice kale and cabbage now and then, and we did love adding apples to just about everything, but by and large our staples were carrot and celery. And so it went.

Mind you, we did love the juice, and we did juice often. But after a while, the juice became a sort of 'oh that' known quantity. We juiced our carrots and celery and apples and we called it good.

Sometime during our second year of juicing, we moved to a new part of the country and as a part of that move, we put in a big garden for the first time in a long time. In many ways, that garden was our juicing salvation, because it shook us out of our rut. But it

34

took a while for us to even realize we had been IN a rut in the first place.

It all started with the cucumbers. We had lots and lots and lots of cucumbers. In fact, we had so many cucumbers we didn't know what to do with them all, and we were way too busy to start making pickles at the time. So we started juicing them.

It was like a revelation! How amazingly delicious are juiced cucumbers? Well, all I can say is you will have to try it to believe it. Especially with a little apple, and maybe half a lemon.

And then there was the chard, and the parsley. The parsley grew to about three feet tall and was just huge. I remembered that when I'd been pregnant with my second child and suffered a bout of anemia my mid-wife had put me on a parsley and orange juice drink I made up in the blender - and so I started juicing the parsley and oranges... Man, what a taste. I could drink that all day long.

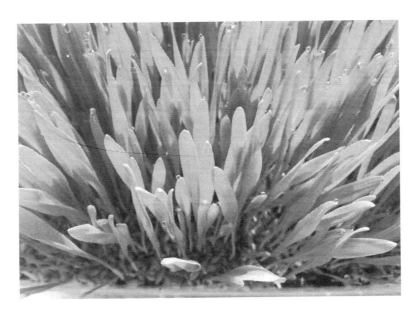

Sometime as all of this was going on, we began growing our own barley grass and adding that to the juices as well. It is very green and very sharp (green) tasting, but if you don't get too crazy with it, it is a great balancer to sweeter fruits and vegetables and it is incredibly good for you.

I still preferred my parsley, but my husband is crazy for barley grass, so I relented.

The lessons here are simple: don't ignore the directions, but don't take them as gospel either. Be willing to experiment within reason. Obviously, if something doesn't fit into the juicing chute, we cut it smaller until it does, but that is really as far as we go. The other lesson? Remember that you are doing something new and don't let yourself get stuck in a rut because you figure out how to do one thing and then never remember to keep trying new things!

Trust me, the more you experiment with your juicer, the happier and more amazed you will be at what it can do and how delicious your new creative inventions can be.

Oh, and speaking of inventions, there's another thing I never did - I never read a juicing recipe until after I had been juicing a few years.

And when I did I was appalled. Who are these people and why do they juice one apple, two carrots and one half a 'beet root'? Personally, if I'm going to juice and drink a juice I make, I want a good 12 ounces or even 16 ounces of juice. I do not count the individual vegetables I juice. I grab a handful of everything, wash it, trim it, and juice it - oh and then I drink it. Just sayin'.

The other thing about this 'juice recipe' thing is that so many of the recipes call for 1/2 this, or 1/2 that - well, I don't need a bunch of half things in my fridge getting spoiled. I know I am normally juicing for two people, but a lot of us are living with at least one other person in our household, so juice accordingly.

When I juice beets, I juice the number of beets in the bunch I bought - usually three. I don't always juice the beet greens, but if I do, I juice them all. Sometimes they are pretty wilted and sad looking, in which case I chop them up and give them to my chickens. If they are gorgeous and firm and yummy, I either juice them or make a salad out of them or do some of both.

One thing I have learned over the years of juicing is that nothing wilts and spoils faster than handfuls of greens left over from juicing sessions - so just juice it - or eat it for lunch in a salad - but don't try to put it away for tomorrow or later in the week. Later in the week it will not be the gorgeous produce it is today. Experience has taught me to make those choices for the best and freshest right now and assume anything left over will be wasted if I don't prepare it, eat it or cook it today.

That is one of the reasons a garden is so amazing. You can go out and pick off exactly the number of kale leaves you want, or chard leaves, or cucumbers, or whatever it is and leave the rest of it all there, still attached to its root mass, still growing, and it will be right there waiting for you tomorrow. At least until the frost comes, but that's another story for another day. For today, just keep playing around with every juicing experience.

And don't expect to get enough juice from one stalk of celery to do much of anything. Buy it by the bunch and use it by the handful of stalks. It's cheap, even organic, and it's incredibly good for you and will give you energy all day.

# Working Out Your Juicing Schedule - How to Juice when Time is short and Days are long

One of the decisions you have to make once you start juicing is whether you will juice every day (or every time you want a fresh juice) or if you are willing to juice and put some of that juice in the refrigerator for later use. It's not a huge decision, but you may find it has a large impact on how often you are having fresh juice.

For us, the answer was and is a moving compromise. There are some weeks when we juice every time we want fresh juice, which is usually every day. But there are other weeks when we juice and store juices in the fridge and only juice two or three times in a week.

There is no question, and I want to be very clear on this, that juices that have just been made are amazing and delicious and beyond anything in the world. There is also no question that a juice you made yesterday is really absolutely incredible even if it is not *quite* as amazing as the fresh one you made yesterday - and that if you had not made it yesterday you would not be drinking it today. Life is full of compromises and choices.

In the world of juicing, it is possible to juice today and drink juice tomorrow and even the next day if that is what it takes to get the job done. It's not perfect, but it is really pretty close.

## Time to Juice: What it takes

When planning a single juicing session for fresh juice to drink now for 1-2 people, you will generally need to budget 15-20 minutes for prep time and juicing, and an additional 10-15 minutes for cleanup. This is a generous time budget, but take your time, especially in the

39

beginning. Unless you're a sous chef, you probably haven't spent a great deal of time preparing produce with a sharp knife. Give yourself time to get the hang of it.

When juicing for multiple days for more than one person, plan to double that amount of time, or approximately one hour from start to finish.

Be sure to read "Specific Instructions for Preparing Your Produce for Juicing" found later in this book in the chapter "Selecting and Preparing Your Produce for Juicing". In general, all produce should be trimmed and then washed before juicing.

## Proper Storage of Juice for later Consumption

There are some strict caveats and guidelines if you are going to juice and store, and you need to know what they are, so you avoid wasting precious fresh fruits and vegetables and time by improperly storing (and thereby ruining) your juices.

The first rule goes back to oxidation; remember only masticating juicers can be used for making juice which can be stored. Additionally, any juice you are going to drink later must be properly sealed and stored in a cold place. Preferably a working refrigerator, but a well-insulated and well-loaded ice chest will do on travel or in a pinch.

The second part of avoiding oxidation of your juices has to do with how full you fill the containers you are storing them in. Each container must be full to the very tippy top. No air space. It must be so full, in fact, that when you open it, you are guaranteed to spill some. That full. No exceptions.

Our solution is to use 12 or 16 ounce mason jars and to use the plastic lids to seal them. (Admittedly, just as in the case of our chopping carrots, it took us a while to figure this out - at first we used the sealing canning jar lids. But we eventually got smart and picked up a few packages of the white plastic mason jar lids and have never looked back. For one thing, you can wash them and re-use them. And, while you can technically re-use the canning jar lids if you are not actually canning with them, they get cruddy and grungy all too soon and you don't WANT to re-use them. So, just start with the white plastic lids and you'll be far happier.)

The jars must be REALLY clean. You do not have to sterilize them as you would for canning, because they will only hold the juice for one to three days maximum. Right, did you get that? Three days maximum. If you haven't taken the juice out and drunk it up in three days then you will be forced to take it out and dump it in the compost. You will know, too, because when you taste it, it will scream "YOU MISSED MY DEADLINE!" and you will not be able to drink it. Trust me on this.

So, run the jars through the dishwasher or wash by hand in hot soapy water and scrub all surfaces. This is particularly true if you are, as we are, re-using them for juice a lot. The juice tends to stick to the glass, and you will need to wash them out with hot water as soon as you empty the jar, so as to avoid build-up of dried-on juice residue.

So, start with your clean mason jars. Fill them to the absolute brim and then seal them up tight and put them in the fridge and you are good for the next 72 hours. Or do it every other day, if that works better for you.

One of the things we do is to juice oranges, lemons and limes or any of the citrus juices separately and put that juice into a quart jar by itself. Then we make up our 12 to 16 ounce veggie juices and mix and match with the orange or citrus juices of our choice when we drink it. Remember just as with the veggie juices to keep your

41

fruit juices full to the brim for the same reason – oxidation will spoil the juice. After you've used some of the citrus juice from the quart jar, transfer the remaining juice to a smaller jar which it fills completely. This will again minimize the air space on top of the juice preventing spoilage.

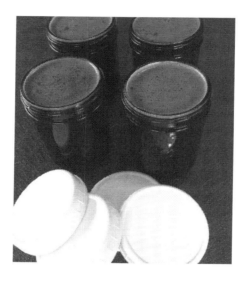

Just pour the veggie juice into a glass and add orange or fruit juices as desired. This is also nice because it means that each person can add as little or as much of the fruit juice to their glass of veggie juice as they like. Custom mixing.

(Right now there is a quart of fresh made orange juice and a quart of fresh made apple juice in our fridge, along with four 16 ounce jars of mixed veggie, herb and root juices.)

When we go on travel the thing we miss the most is our juicer. Even though juicing has become more popular, there are only certain cities around the country where commercial juice bars are common place. And if you can find one, expect to pay upwards of $10 for a single juice.

So, if we are traveling by car, we'll bring along enough juice for two days in a well packed cooler. That means the cooler has a seriously full load of ice in it and we re-fill that ice if we expect to have juice the second day. It can be done. But if the cooler gets warm, or things go haywire, don't drink the juice.

The good thing about these fresh juices is, if something has gone wrong in keeping it cool, you will not need a scientist to tell you not to drink it. You will open it and even one tiny taste will tell you - and, even if you take that tiny taste, it won't hurt you. It just won't taste good. Now, if you drink it anyway, I cannot tell you if it will hurt you, I've never been that stubborn.

## Keeping Control of Your Juicing Budget

One of the trickiest things about buying fresh produce is learning how much is enough and how much is too much. Nothing puts a kink in your budget like throwing out produce that has spoiled before you get to use it; and it's a very common experience.

As juicers, we can solve some of this problem by juicing what is on hand before it spoils, but there are some important things to know about buying and storing fresh produce nonetheless.

In the old days of small villages and local shops, people went to the green grocer a few times a week and didn't have to worry about storing produce for any longer than a couple of days at a time. But these days, we often end up shopping only once a week, and have to plan carefully what we need in order not to run out of fresh produce and not to be throwing something away uneaten because it has spoiled.

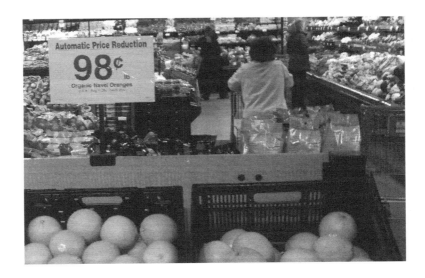

Unfortunately, for a large majority of us, frozen and canned foods became the norm for a number of decades after the advent of flash freezing methods; particularly in the U.S. While we still purchased fresh fruits and salad vegetables, many households spent very little of their food budget in the produce aisle.

The lack of experience with shopping for fresh produce can become an obstacle in itself. We literally do not know how to store produce or even what some of it is! One of our favorite resources for produce education is Mark Mulcahy, co-host of the radio show "An Organic Conversation" which broadcasts out of San Francisco every Saturday. It is also available on their website (http://www.anorganicconversation.com/) and as a podcast on iTunes.

One of the interesting things we learned from listening to Mark, for instance, is that we should not wash our strawberries or other delicate berry fruits until we are ready to use them. We were very happy to learn this one, because we had lost a lot of beautiful berries, even from our own gardens, by doing it wrong. As soon as they are washed they start to break down. For instance, we would pick a nice big bowl of strawberries from the garden, bring them in and wash them. Even when stored in the fridge, by the end of the day, or early the next day, they were beginning to become mushy, and within a few days they would develop mold. What a sad fate for such beautiful fruits! Now we don't make that mistake anymore, and our berries last quite nicely for more than several days in the fridge, because they are dry. We wash them just before we eat or juice them, and never earlier.

Another tip we learned from Mark Mulcahy was to keep our peaches and nectarines on the counter. Often when you buy peaches and nectarines, they are still hard and will need a few days to ripen. The thing is, once they start to ripen, they all ripen at once. But, as Mark pointed out, and it is completely true, once you put either of these fruits in the refrigerator they lose their amazing flavor almost instantly and it doesn't come back. So only buy as many as you can eat in a couple of days even if they are not ripe yet, and then when they do ripen you won't be throwing out the ones you cannot eat fast enough. Of course if you are juicing, you can juice them up and have the juice for a couple more days, so long as the juice is stored properly.

Another great idea we use every summer is to freeze whole peaches on a cookie sheet just as you would blueberries or strawberries. Wait until they are ripe but not over ripe. Lay them out on the cookie sheet on a sheet of freezer paper and freeze them solid - usually overnight is all it takes. Don't leave them in longer than necessary to freeze solid, or they can develop freezer burn.

Once they are frozen, bag them in Ziploc® freezer bags, removing as much air as possible. A drinking straw inserted as you close the bag can be used to suck out as much air as possible as you zip the bag closed and slip the straw out. It takes a little practice to get it just right but it works like a charm once you get the knack.

This is a great way to save peaches and nectarines when the season is in full swing and prices are low. You can use them as frozen fruit desserts later in the year - and your Omega Juicer can be used to make them, too!

You can also simply remove the frozen fruits from the freezer and run them under warm water to gently thaw, and make excellent peach pies, sauces and smoothies with them.

We keep bags of whole frozen peaches, nectarines and blueberries in the freezer and pull them out for smoothies, frozen desserts, pie and muffin baking all winter and right up to the next harvest the following summer. Nothing like fresh blueberry pancakes any time you want them for a special Sunday breakfast.

The best thing about using this method of buying in season and freezing is that you have excellent additions for fresh juices all year long at bargain prices. We buy organic peaches for around 90 cents a pound in August when the crop hits full swing. Otherwise they can often run 2 to 3 dollars a pound. That's a big savings for your budget.

If you do want to juice them after they've been frozen, let them thaw on the counter for a few hours. Blueberries can also be juiced this way, although you will get less juice from them than you will from fresh. We tend to use the blueberries for the frozen desserts with the juicer, rather than for fresh juice.

## Juicing Staples

You can certainly pick up carrots and celery most times of the year because both of these crops are grown year round in green houses all over the place. Carrots are a root crop which means they are generally plentiful all fall and winter, and if they get slim, look for yams as an additional sweet and orange replacement in the short term.

Beets are also more and more commonly found throughout a large part of the year, and the natural organic bunch beets are often selling at 2 bunches for $5 in our part of the world. You can juice the whole thing, greens and all. Or you can chop off the greens' tops and make a salad or put them in soups and stews.

Produce even when organic, is not that expensive if you know where and when to shop. In comparison, processed and packaged foods continue to rise dramatically in price.

The increased demand for fresh organic produce has also expanded its availability. For instance, Costco sells a good selection of organic produce at very reasonable prices these days. One of their large boxes of organic baby spinach goes for around $4. That is often half of what specialty grocers will be charging for the same product.

## Storing Produce

Sweet potatoes, apples, oranges, lemons, limes and pears all have a relatively flexible at-home storage time of five to ten days. This makes them all good juicing material that can be used several times over a week without having to worry about spoiling. Apples and pears can be stored in the refrigerator in between layers of freezer paper for up to three months depending on their type. Sweet potatoes can be kept on a counter or in a cool dark cupboard just as you would store a potato or an onion. Citrus will need refrigeration after about five days depending on your indoor climate, as they can develop mold.

When it comes to fresh greens, your timing must be a bit more precise and these must be kept refrigerated. Herbs, greens, lettuces, and other tender-leaved vegetables are all more susceptible to spoiling, and so should be used within a few days of purchase.

Happily, these tender greens are also some of the easiest things to grow, and having a nice crop of fresh greens in a sunny spot in the window, on a patio or deck in warm weather is really a snap. You don't need a whole kitchen garden but if you are so inclined it will save you even more on your juicing budget.

Here is a typical week's supply of juicing materials around our house. We are two people, but we generally drink a 12 to 16 ounce juice per person per day, so that should give you a good idea of what to expect to need once you become a regular juicer:

Carrots: 2 to 4 pounds, we usually buy two 2lb bags once a week, with some weeks only needing one as there are some left from the week before.

Beets: 2 bunches of beets with 3 to 4 beets each including greens.

Celery: 2 nice large bunches.

Oranges, Apples, Pears: We tend to rotate these around depending on the season. In winter we buy more oranges as they are in season and also contain the extra vitamin C to help us stay healthy and ward off colds and flu. 4 to 6 oranges, apples or pears or a mix of all three.

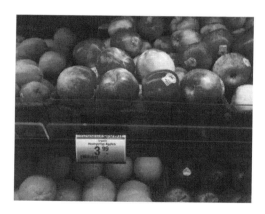

Ginger: A good sized piece of ginger root will last a month, just keep it in the fridge wrapped in a bit of cellophane. In fact, it will last longer if all you use it for is juicing. All you need is a 1 inch piece for a juice session making 2 to 4 large juices. Ginger is potent and should always be added into the juice earlier rather than later. It will sit on the top of the finished juice if added too late. If juiced last, it will mostly end up staying in the juicer and never get into your juice. Some people are sensitive to ginger, so please test for taste and increase in small increments.

We also juice cabbages, kale, chard, and green lettuces and spinach. These we also rotate over the seasons depending on price, availability, and seasonality. Lettuce can get to $3 a head in deep winter, while kale and cabbages tend to be cheaper this time of year. One cabbage, one Swiss chard or one kale or any two of any of the greens should be plenty for a week's worth of juicing.

Parsley, cilantro, basil, fennel, arugula and mint all make excellent additions to fresh juices and the best way to determine which to use is to try them all a little bit at a time mixed in to your juices. We are huge fans of curly parsley in juices, both for the iron and for the taste. Parsley adds a really pleasant zing to a veggie juice and is particularly tasty with a little citrus in the mix.

## Example of a Weekly Juicing Budget

So here is our weekly budget for juicing, to help you get an idea of what can be done at what price. Do remember that the best juice is one you actually make and drink, and all the beautiful fresh produce in the world will only go bad if you don't stick to your plans and break out the juicer and make the juice. Because this is a new routine, it helps to set a plan and budget and stick to it for a couple of weeks or even months so that you develop the habit of juicing on a regular basis. Otherwise you may find your good intentions lead to lots of produce purchasing and not enough juicing; which will lead to a lot of wasted produce and bad feelings about not keeping up with your plan or your produce. And of course, the prices shown here represent a snapshot in time for our region.

| Organic Carrots | Two 2lb-bags | $3.00 |
|---|---|---|
| Organic Celery | 2 large bunches (2 lbs.) | $4.00 |
| Organic Cabbage, green or red | 2 to 3 lbs. | $5.00 |
| Organic Cucumber | 1 large | $2.00 |
| Organic Beets | 2 bunches of 3 beets each with greens | $5.00 |
| Organic Apples and Pears | 3 | $5.00 |
| Organic Oranges | 3 | $3.00 |
| Organic Lemons | 2 | $2.00 |
| Organic Greens (spinach, lettuce, chard, kale, collard greens, etc.) | 2 bunches or 1 lb.-box of organic baby spinach | $5.00 |
| Organic Sweet Potatoes | 2 to 3 | $3.00 |
| Organic Barley Grass | home grown from seed | $1.00 |
| Organic Herbs (Parsley etc.) | 1 bunch | $2.00 |
| Organic Ginger | 2 or 3 small (1-inch long) pieces | $1.00 |
| Organic Turmeric | 2 or 3 small (1-inch long) root pieces | $1.00 |
| Specialty Items In Season (basil, mint, parsley, fennel, etc.) | 1 bunch | $3.00 |

Total weekly budget: $45.00

## CSA's and Farmers Markets - Another Big Budget Saver

A great way to save on fresh produce in season and to have a steady supply of excellent locally grown organic juicing materials is to shop through a local CSA or Farmers Market.

CSA's are "Community Supported Agriculture" programs where local farms allow you to purchase an annual subscription based on a weekly cost and receive fresh produce each week during the growing season. Some CSA farms deliver; others have pick-up days for customers at the farm or at a convenient in-town location. Each farm handles their program slightly differently, so you'll want to check around and choose the farm and program that works best for you.

Until very recently, CSA's were not a very common option for most people throughout the U.S. and around the world. But that has changed dramatically in the last decade and in the last few years. CSA's have exploded as farmers and consumers discover that direct relationships work well for everyone involved.

> ⇒ TIP: To find a local CSA in your area, the best resource is a web site called Local Harvest. You can find them at http://localharvest.org and they have a complete directory of local farms, CSA's, Farmers Markets and even allow you to search by specific products you are looking for. They have a nationwide database search engine and it is very good.

Another way to find local CSAs is to look up local community food and farmers markets and speak with the people who run them and to the farmers who sell at the markets. Often local farms have a

CSA and a farmers market program, so you can find a farm selling the produce you like at the farmers market and inquire if they run a CSA as well.

So don't let anyone tell you that it is 'too expensive to eat organic'. It is only too expensive if you insist on buying everything cello-wrapped at the local national chain store. And even then, if you shop wisely and in season, it is cheaper sometimes by half or more than it will be the rest of the year.

Learning how to move your purchasing power around with the seasons and varying your juicing and produce consumption over the course of the year can drastically reduce what you spend.

# Selecting and Preparing Your Produce for Juicing

## Produce Selection and Seasonality

As you get into the habit of juicing you will learn more and more about the nature of the produce you juice. You will learn that in different seasons and from different sources, produce tastes differently! Sometimes a certain vegetable will be incredibly sweet, sometimes more hot and pungent. Just as any experienced vegetable gardener knows, different temperatures, moisture and weather conditions directly affect the taste of the produce you grow. This does not change simply because you are buying your produce in the local shop or grocery store. A large part of produce selection is variable and has to do with seasons, climate and growing conditions.

For most of us, selecting produce at the grocery store seems a fairly predictable and mundane task, but that is simply because we are disconnected from the immediacy of the growing phenomenon. Selecting the best produce for juicing is highly dependent on season. Getting to learn the natural seasons of your produce will give you a big advantage when it comes to selecting the best juicing materials as you move through the seasons.

One of the most important and simple rules of juicing is to taste the produce you are juicing as you go! In our household we jokingly say "That's eating the juicing material, isn't it?!", and the answer is always YES. Because if you do not taste it as it goes into the juicer you do not know what it will taste like coming OUT of the juicer. The answer is, it will always taste even more powerfully of whatever it tastes like going in. So a 'hot' cabbage or a sweet Kale will taste hot or sweet in the juice. Some seasons, kale is so sweet it is like candy, others it is so bitter it is like coffee. Knowing how it tastes going in helps you balance the juice so that it is delicious and palatable coming out of the juicer and into your glass.

There will be juices where you will look at your mate or friend or juicing partner and say "WOW that is AMAZING!" and there will be juices where you take one sip and say "Where is the apple/orange/lemon/yam/beet (fill in the blank) to make this juice drinkable!?!"

So, rule number one when preparing your juices, is to TASTE the produce you are juicing. A little nibble is all it takes to know - bitter? sweet? pleasant? super-astringent? Makes your hair stand up on end? It is completely worth the tiny effort it takes to nibble as you juice and it will pay you back in spades. Every once in a while you will nibble and say "YECH! P.U., ACK!" and because you will be in the midst of making a delicious juice, you will refrain from adding that YECH to your juice before it is too late and you have spoiled a perfectly lovely juice.

This is the reality of juicing. You cannot 'taste test' every piece of produce you buy, so you learn to taste test as you juice. It is so worth it. It will also teach you a valuable long term vocabulary of tastes in the produce world that will serve you well as you go on to develop your juicing regimen over the long term. No one says you have to juice any particular vegetable or fruit to be a successful juicer and if you determine that something doesn't work for you then you can simply eliminate it early on and not have to worry about it.

That being said, the other thing you will discover over time is that your taste will change when it comes to juices and juicing. So every once in a while, go ahead and go back and experiment with that thing you decided was never going to be in your juice again - you may just surprise yourself.

Rule number two for selecting produce is to go organic when at all possible. This is particularly important for the produce on the infamous 'dirty dozen' list of most highly toxic from pesticides, which include quite a few of the most popularly juiced fruits and vegetables. Those familiar with produce will most likely know these, but just in case there is any question in your mind, here they are again:

Apples
Celery
Strawberries
Peaches
Spinach
Nectarines
Grapes (esp. imported grapes)
Sweet bell peppers
Potatoes
Blueberries
Lettuce
Kale (tie)
Collard Greens (tie)

These items have been tested and rated for pesticide residue by the Environmental Working Group as of the 2010 harvest (testing completed in 2011) and are the produce items most heavily loaded with pesticide residue. The last thing you need to be doing when you juice is adding pesticide residue to your diet. So, if you cannot buy these products as organic, the best idea is to skip them altogether, or grow your own.

The importance of this list is twofold. First, you need to know where you are most likely to encounter high levels of toxic chemicals in your food. Second, you need to know which foods are particularly excellent juicing candidates and so highly nutritious that they should be in your juicing regimen.  In the list above, the items that jump out as important members of that list are apples, celery, blueberries, kale and collard greens. These are all excellent cleansing foods (isn't that ironic?) and eliminating them from your juicing regimen would be a serious loss.  One way to solve this problem is to look for them at local farmers markets and be sure to ask the sellers if they do not specifically state that their produce is organic.  Another solution is to frequent local grocers who carry a larger selection of organic produce. Here in the Pacific Northwest that means local smaller grocery chains such as Market of Choice, or even the regional chain, Fred Meyer where there is a much higher assortment of both local and organic produce than in many of the nationwide chain stores.

So don't give up too soon if you don't find the organic produce you want for juicing right away. You can often find it, and it does not have to be super expensive either. See the chapter on planning your juicing budget for more tips on best shopping practices for your produce for juicing.

There are also what is known as the 'Clean 15' which are the produce items with the LOWEST measured pesticide residue for the same period.  I'm not sure why the newer 2011 harvest data results don't seem to be showing up anywhere yet, but perhaps they are so similar, the folks at the Environmental Working Group didn't think they needed to re-do the list.

Here is their 2011 Clean 15 list:

1. Onions
2. Sweet Corn
3. Pineapple
4. Avocado
5. Asparagus
6. Sweet peas

7. Mango
8. Eggplant
9. Cantaloupe (domestic)
10. Kiwi
11. Cabbage
12. Watermelon
13. Sweet Potatoes
14. Grapefruit
15. Mushrooms

Unfortunately, not all of these are great for juicing - but a lot of them are. The cantaloupe and kiwi, and of course cabbage; and adding a grapefruit to your citrus mix can jazz things up nicely as well. Sweet potatoes (aka yams), mango, asparagus and pineapple are all perfectly good juicing candidates.

## Specific Instructions for Preparing Your Produce for Juicing

We know, it's true, the manual for the Omega juicer says to chop everything into small pieces in order to extract the maximum amount of juice; but, honestly, it is not necessary and it takes way too much time. Refer to our newbie juicer mistakes chapter here.

There are some things you can do to make juicing quick and easy and to get the most out of your juicing produce and chopping them all into small pieces is not one of them.

So here are the steps to take to prepare your produce for juicing, in alphabetical order to keep it simple and easy:

Apples: Wash, core and juice. Do not juice the core. Do not peel. Larger apples will need to be cut across the cored sections to make them narrow enough to fit into the juicing chute.

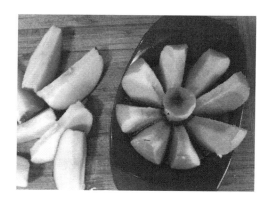

Beets: Scrub well with a vegetable brush. Cut off root tail and cut greens just below the leaf. Cut lengthwise into pieces slender enough to fit into the chute. Juice greens separately from the beets using celery, carrots or other firm vegetables to help feed them through the juicer. Or keep the leaves aside for salads, soups and stews.

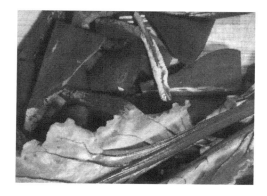

Bananas: You cannot juice fresh bananas, too mushy, but you can freeze them and use the blank cap and make great banana ice desserts. Cut the banana into lengthwise pieces before you freeze it.

Barley Grass: Cut sections two inches square out of your growing container and feed into juicer in small bunches with firm vegetables or fruit to help feed them in and get them all through the juicer. Barley grass is very astringent, so only use one two inch square of grass at a time (about 6 to 10 inches tall) until you get used to the taste or decide you want more.

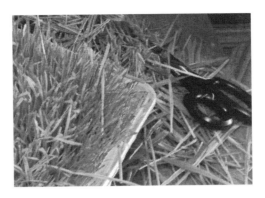

Basil: rinse a handful of leaves and either shake or pat dry. Basil is quite pungent fresh, delicious, but start by adding just a few leaves at a time and add more to taste. Wonderful with cucumber and half a lemon.

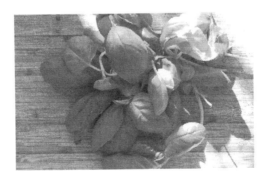

Bok Choy:  For small heads, separate outer leaves and wash thoroughly as they may have dirt trapped along the base. Inner leaves of the head are usually clean enough for just a quick rinse. Chop lengthwise to 3/4 inch widths. For large heads, cut the bottom half inch of the base off before washing and proceed as above. Very light and refreshing taste, great with apple and celery.

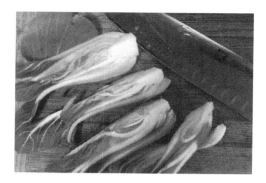

Broccoli: Wash and shake to remove excess water from floret heads. Cut off base of stem and cut whole stalks lengthwise to fit into juicer chute. Great with half a lemon or lime.

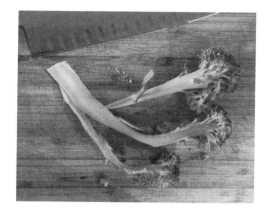

Cabbage: Remove outer leaves, usually two or three leaves will get the outer surface fully removed. Cut in half and then cut 'wedges' about 1/2 inch thick. Break apart wedges to get slender enough sections to feed into the chute. Cabbages can be surprising - some are super sweet and some are hot and spicy. Taste the cabbage as you juice it to determine which it is and how much of it you want in your juice.

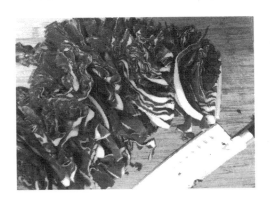

Carrots: Cut off stem ends first, then scrub well with a vegetable brush. For large carrots cut lengthwise to make them into skinny sticks, for small or medium carrots juice whole.

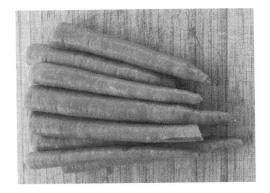

Celery: Cut off base of stalks and trim any wilted leaves, then scrub with a vegetable brush. For larger stalks, break lengthwise by squeezing the outer edges toward the middle so they will fit into the chute.

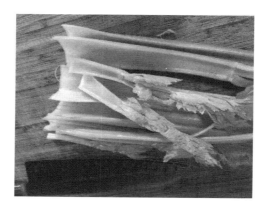

Chard: Wash and shake excess water off leaves. Remove any wilted or spoiled spots and feed into juicer either leaf tip or stem first. Chard is generally sturdy enough to be fed into the juicer either way. Use a carrot or celery to 'push' it through the juicer.

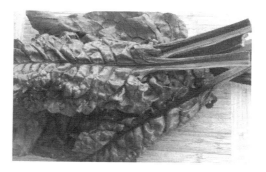

Chives: wash and shake dry, use small bunches at a time and slide into the juicer, use a carrot or celery stick to push them in and help get them through the juicer.

Citrus: All citrus are great in juices. The best way to prepare them is to cut just through the peel in a complete circumference of the fruit, then turn 90 degrees and cut again all the way around so that you have four sections of peel from top to bottom that can be easily peeled off without puncturing the cells of the fruit. Once peeled, simply slide in your finger and separate the sections and juice them whole. This keeps more of the juice in the fruit until it gets into the juicer and wastes less juice which is typically lost when you cut the citrus up into pieces. There is something amazing about a juice of orange, lemon and lime - really complex and delicious tasting.

We like to juice four or five oranges, a lemon and a lime or some combination of them all and then set that juice in its own mason jar and add it to taste to our veggie juices as we drink them.

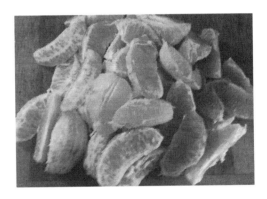

Cress: Water and land cress are both great powerhouses of nutrition and excellent in juices. They are on the peppery - hot side, so mix them with carrot, beet or yam to mellow the peppery flavor.

Cucumber: Cucumbers are generally available either waxed or unwaxed. If you grow your own or buy from local farmers they are generally unwaxed. Grocery store cukes are often waxed. This matters because if they are waxed you need to peel them. (You don't want to juice wax and drink it!) If you are unsure, peel them. Cucumbers can also be bitter at their ends. To avoid bitterness either routinely cut off their ends or make sure to taste test before you add them to the juice. Then cut them lengthwise into quarters so they are slender enough to go down the chute. Sometimes if they are really fat and round you will need to cut them again before they will fit. They make a delicious and extremely healthy juice and add a light and delicious flavor to any other produce juice combination. One of our favorites.

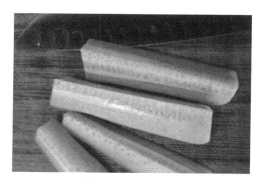

Dandelion: Juice the leaves and not the root. The root can be made into a delicious tea, but is best brewed. Wash and shake leaves and insert into chute in small bunches. Dandelion is potent, so use a little bit at a time and taste before adding more!

Fennel: Wash and shake dry. Cut lengthwise from the top, separating out the individual stalks as you go. Some of these will still be too wide at the base for juicing, cut the base bulb down to more slender pieces. Fennel is surprisingly mild and wonderful in a raw juice. It is also incredibly good for you. Wait for it to come into season (winter/early spring) and get it at the best prices. Delicious!

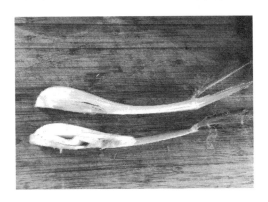

Garlic: Peel and juice individual cloves. Use it sparingly. It is very pungent and powerful when juiced raw. We do not juice garlic often, preferring to add it to cooked foods or to roast whole garlic heads and enjoy the more mild roasted flavor.

Ginger: Cut off a one inch section of root and peel. Juice ginger while juicing carrots, yams, celery, apples or other firm fruit as it needs to be 'pushed' through the juicer for the best effect. Ginger is quite pungent and some people 'feel' it in their sinuses when they drink it in a raw juice. I personally love it and have no problem with this, but test it for yourself to find the right amount. Usually one 1-inch piece of peeled root is plenty for a juice session for one or two people.

Kale: Wash and shake to remove excess water. For extra large leaves, cut lengthwise and feed into chute leafy top first, using the stem to help to push the rest through. Kale is one of our favorites for juicing. It is astringent, but it is also truly delicious. In the right season (cool weather early spring and/or fall crops, it is incredibly sweet. We find ourselves eating the leaves as we juice so that half of it is eaten during the juicing process and the rest gets into the juice. In late spring and summer kale can become suddenly super bitter if the heat has come on before the harvest, so taste it and temper the amounts if it is bitter. It is still good in the juice when bitter, but too much will really give you that sense of drinking a juice that is good for you rather than good tasting.

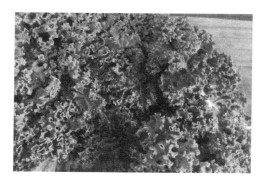

Lettuce: Wash and shake off excess water, cut length-wise to make slender strips. Some lettuce is hardier/more firm than others, for the more delicate leaves, use a celery stalk or carrot to help clear it through the juicer. Lettuce is a lovely light flavor and very high in water volume like spinach, so it gives a nice volume of juice for its mass that is light and pleasant tasting.

Lemon: As with all citrus, the best way to prepare lemons for juicing is to use a paring knife and cut through the skin only (as much as possible) in a circumference around the whole fruit and then do that again off-set by 90 degrees. This will give you a fruit with the skin cut into quarters and the fruit un-cut. Gently peel away the rind of each quarter section until all the peel is removed. Then carefully separate into section pieces which will fit into the chute. This method will allow you to separate the citrus into small enough sections for the juicer without actually breaking open the juice containing cells of the fruit.

Melon: Cut and remove seeds and cut into wedges. Some melons are so large that it is easiest to cut the wedges into juicer sized pieces. For smaller melons, simply cut the wedges and then remove the melon peel and drop whole wedges into the chute. Melon is another of the lovely high water content light flavor options to lighten and sweeten high greens content juices.

Mint: Mint is a great addition to most juices. You don't need much. One bunch of mint can last through a whole week's worth of juices. Just a few sprigs is all you need to brighten up any juice.

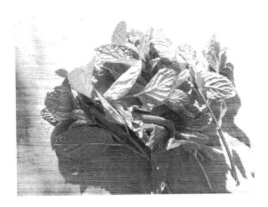

Parsley: One of our all-time favorites for juicing, we are generous with the parsley and have no trouble adding half a good sized bunch to one juice. We just love the stuff. It is also very high in iron and adding any citrus to a juice with parsley in it will give your body instant access to the iron while boosting your calcium intake.

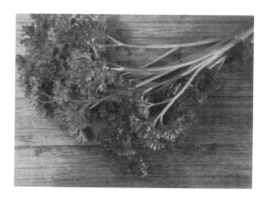

Radish: Another hot and peppery one, you can use daikon or red 'breakfast' radishes. The small red ones are sweet in season and won't make the juice too peppery, but taste them first, because once hot weather hits, they tend to get more peppery tasting. We like using three or four of the young cool weather variety in our regular juices. Once summer comes, we cut it down to one or two and use the rest of them in salads and sandwiches. One bunch of radishes can last all week.

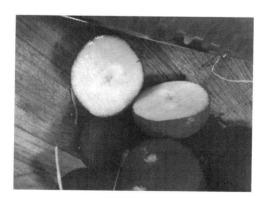

Spinach: This is another one that can be used anytime and because it is grown in greenhouses all over the country, it's relatively easy to find. Pre-washed organic baby leaves are the highest in nutritive value and the easiest to juice. Just add a small handful at a time and push them through with a carrot, celery or other firmer vegetable to help push them through the juicer.

Sweet Potatoes: Sweet Potatoes (Yams) are the other sweet vegetable when it comes to juicing. Use them to temper super green drinks or for an amazing winter treat with carrot, celery, beets and a little mint or parsley. Also excellent as a juice with orange.

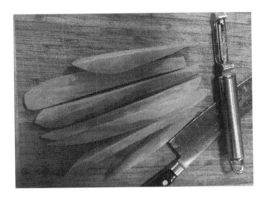

Tomato: A great summer juicing vegetable. Cut into wedges slender enough to fit in the juicer chute and juice away. Excellent with celery and parsley and lemon or lime.

Turnips: Wash and cut into pieces that will fit into the chute.

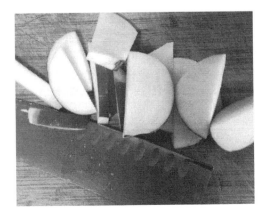

Yams: See Sweet Potatoes.

# Benefits of Juicing - The Ingredients to Get the Results You Want

This section will give you hands on tips for preparing your fruits, veggies and herbs for juicing as well as give you some examples of juices you can make, and get you started on your own exploration of mixing and matching juicing ingredients.

While I've never been a big fan of specific juice recipes, I am a big fan of knowing the ingredients that work best to achieve my desired result. It's not hard to find lots of recipes for juicing out there; and it's a simple thing to compare a lot of different people's ideas of recipes and begin to see how they all work together - which ingredients do what, and so forth.

➡ TIPS:

Always peel all citrus before juicing.
Use all organic vegetables whenever possible.
Trim Carrot tops and Celery roots/base.
Trim all vegetables as needed before washing.
Use a vegetable brush and wash all ingredients well before juicing.
Core Apples and Pears before juicing.
Cucumbers with wax coatings should be peeled. No wax? No peeling needed.
Cucumbers can have bitter ends; remove ends or taste for bitterness before juicing.
Always juice soft/greens/leafy items first and hard items last (Carrots make a great last item to help clean out the juicer.)
Always wash the juicer IMMEDIATELY after use.

Each of us has to gauge what works best for us individually, but we also have to go through a period of discovery.  Try not to back yourself into a corner or fall into a rut of only juicing one way or at one time of day or even with only certain ingredients.

Use the Juicing Ingredients Guide in the next chapter to get detailed nutritional information on a wide variety of vegetables, fruits and herbs to help guide your juicing ingredient choices.

## Detox Juices

These are the juices that help your body flush out toxins and restore vitality. Most of us do not do nearly enough regular cleansing to help our bodies stay clean on the inside. Increasing our clean water intake, regular exercise, stretching and a regular practice of receiving massages can all aid in getting our detoxification system back in order. You will see and feel these changes quickly if you give your body a chance to get clean. The fastest way to do that is to stop putting in food or anything else other than juices and clean water for a few days, or even a few weeks if you can do it. Otherwise, start by replacing your first meal of the day with these juices - your results will not be as quick to materialize, but they will be just as dramatic as they do.

*Greens and Cleansing Veggies:*
- Barley Grass
- Celery
- Cilantro
- Cucumber
- Dandelion
- Kale
- Parsley
- Spinach
- Swiss Chard
- Wheatgrass

*Balancing Veggies:*
- Beets
- Carrots
- Sweet Potato

*Fruits:*

- Apples
- Cantaloupe
- Kiwi
- Lemon
- Lime
- Oranges
- Pears

*Optional Extra Power Boosters:*

- Ginger
- Turmeric

You can mix and match these ingredients for great detoxifying juices with the understanding that the main purpose of the detox juice is to get those greens and astringent veggies to work for you without too much sweet. Here are some standard combinations for detoxing juices.

| |
|---|
| 1 Cantaloupe and 2 to 3 Kiwi |
| 1 bunch Parsley, 2 stalks Celery, 1 bunch Cilantro, 1 Lemon (peeled), 1 inch fresh Ginger |
| 1 bunch Parsley, 3 stalks Celery, 3 Carrots, 2 Apples |
| 1 bunch Parsley, 4 large leaves Swiss Chard, 1 Cucumber, 2 stalks Celery, 1 Green Apple, 1 Lemon |
| 1 Cucumber, 3 stalks Celery, 1 Bunch Barley Grass, 1 Lemon |
| 2 cups Swiss Chard, 1 cup Kale, 3 Carrots, 2 stalks Celery, 2 green Apples |

Feel free to add handfuls of any of the greens in the first list to any juice for added cleansing power.

One of our favorite super boosting detox drinks is Food Babe's Romaine, Cucumber, Turmeric and Lemon 'Cooler' - it's very zippy and refreshing and the Turmeric is incredibly good for you.

## Losing-Weight Juices

The easiest way to lose weight with juicing is to replace one meal a day with a fresh juice to start. See how that goes for you and, if you want to, increase to two meals a day. Drink plenty of clean water, and try to get out and move your body, even a simple daily walk can do the trick.

Juices high in the cleansing greens like chard and parsley and mineral-rich body-supporting greens like spinach will help your body support the weight loss without fatigue or draining of your nutritional reserves. Another important thing to remember about weight gain in these modern times is that many doctors attribute excess weight to toxicity levels in the body tissues and blood, so a good cleansing detox juice is very supportive of weight loss juicing.

*Greens:*
- Chard
- Spinach
- Parsley

*Balancing Veggies:*
- Carrot
- Celery
- Cucumber

*Fruits:*
- Apple
- Kiwi
- Lemon
- Pear

Pears, apples, lemons and greens are all great for helping the body cleanse and lose weight. Cucumbers and celery add a lightness and provide important nutrients to keep you healthy as you go. Kiwi, carrot and parsley boost your vitamin C and beta-carotene.

1 bunch Parsley, 2 Celery stalks, 1 Cucumber, 1 Green Pear, 1/2 Lemon
2 cups Spinach, 2 Carrots, 2 Celery stalks, 1 Apple
3 large leaves Swiss Chard, 2 Carrots, 1 Apple, 1 Lemon

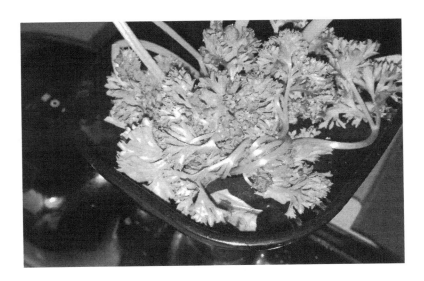

## Looking-Younger Juices

These are the ingredients which give your skin that super healthy glow, reduce wrinkles and give you the support within your whole body to energize and feel the power of your younger stronger self.

*Veggies:*
- Celery
- Carrots
- Cucumber
- Green Pepper
- Parsley

*Fruits:*
- Apple
- Blueberries
- Lemon
- Tomatoes

*Optional Extra Power Boosters*
- Aloe Vera

Cucumber has long been known as a skin rejuvenator, either directly on the skin or by drinking. When possible buy organic un-waxed cucumbers so that you can juice the skins as well. Carrot will provide UV protection as well as giving your skin a healthy beta-carotene glow. Tomatoes are high in lycopene which has also recently been shown to be important in bone health. Maintaining healthy bones helps you maintain good posture and balance, keeping you young.

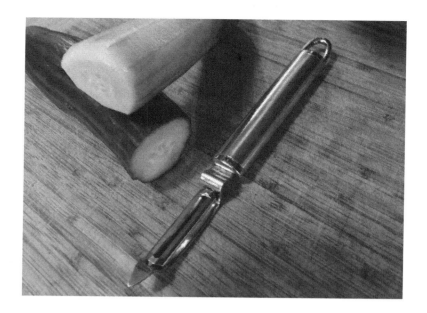

Here are some examples of how to mix and match to get you started:

2 Apples, 3 cups fresh or thawed frozen Blueberries
1 Cucumber, 2 Celery stalks, 3 Carrots, 1 Apple
3 Tomatoes, 2 Celery stalks, 2 Carrots, 1 bunch Parsley
2 Tomatoes, 1 Cucumber, 1 small Green Pepper, 1/2 Lemon

Again, remember you can mix and match to taste as long as you keep a balance between fruits and vegetables. In the case of blueberries, their antioxidant properties are very high and they are less sweet than most berries. They also help improve memory, so you can remember how great you look!

## Immunity Booster Juices

These are the juices to ward off colds and flu, increase stamina and give you that extra oomph, especially needed in the winter when people around you are sneezing and coughing and you do not want to join them. Some of them are pure Vitamin C bombs, others mix it up a bit. In any event, they will do the job of giving you the extra fire power you need to stay on your game and not go down for the count.

*Veggies:*
- Barley Grass
- Celery
- Carrot

*Fruits:*
- Apple
- Grapefruit
- Kiwi
- Orange
- Pear

*Optional Extra Power Boosters:*
- Ginger
- Onion
- Garlic

Ginger, garlic and onion all have antibacterial properties to help clean out your system. Grapefruit, Kiwi, Orange and Lemon give you the super doses of Vitamin C to boost the whole immune function. Carrots add the essential beta-carotene to help the body utilize all that goodness.

1 medium Grapefruit, 1 medium Orange, 2 to 4 Kiwis

1 small Onion, 2 cloves Garlic, 1 one-inch piece Ginger, 3 Oranges, 1 Lemon, handful of Parsley

1 small bunch of Barley Grass, 2 Carrots, 4 stalks Celery, 1 Apple, 1 Lemon, 1 Lime, 2 small pieces of Ginger

1 green Pear, 1 green Apple, 2 stalks Celery, 3 Carrots, 1 small bunch of Barley Grass, 1 clove Garlic, 1 one-inch piece of Ginger, 1 Lemon

Are you starting to see the overlap here? The truth is, yes, all of these juices do the things they are designed to do in these groupings, but they all do so much of everything that any juicing you do is going to be so good for your overall health, you'll notice it in all of these effects.

Healthy looking skin, shiny hair, strong nails, normalized weight, increased energy and improved memory all come along with improved energy and stamina and a general sense of increased well-being.

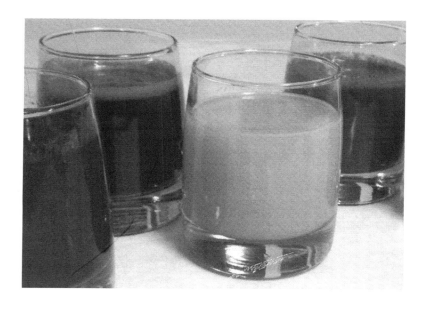

# Vitamins, Minerals, Produce and Juicing - Making the Connection for Better Health

Vitamins and minerals are two of the major building blocks when it comes to the operating system of the human body. Together they provide the energy exchange and cellular nutrition functions which run all systems. These systems allow us to see properly, build strong bones, blood, organs, muscles, cell walls, vascular systems and everything else that our bodies do to keep us functioning. They regulate our blood pressure, insulin and blood sugar levels, blood clotting and thinning and internal acid/base balance.

Vitamins and minerals work together to give us all the essential components of our enzyme, amino acid and cell, bone, blood, tissue and organ support systems.

The trick to their proper functioning is that they cannot accomplish the complex tasks of building all the internal systems which run our bodies without each other. Vitamins without certain minerals cannot be utilized by our bodies, no matter how much of the vitamin is provided.

While it is true that modern nutritional science goes far beyond vitamins and minerals into such complex systems as phytochemicals and accessory nutrients, it all starts with these two partners, vitamins and minerals, if we are to maintain good health.

The power of juicing really shines when we look at intake of vitamins and minerals for two reasons. First, we can juice the equivalent of many servings of fruits and vegetables and consume them as one juice, with a very low relative caloric intake and a super-high nutritional density.

Second, we can juice much larger quantities of certain herbs and vegetables than we would otherwise normally eat.

Parsley is an excellent example of this. In most nutritional analysis, parsley is measured in tablespoon amounts. 2 tablespoons of parsley provide 3% of the daily intake of folate, for example. But one cup of parsley contains the full 100 percent of the daily intake amount, and is easy and delicious to add to any juice. The same is true for iron in parsley. Additionally, fresh herbs are loaded with volatile oils which make them particularly potent healing foods, so juicing one bunch of cilantro, parsley, or a handful of mint or basil along with your veggies and fruits adds a significant healing boost to your diet.

## Vitamins

Vitamins can be broken into two groups:

- Fat-soluble vitamins: A, D, E and K
- Water-soluble vitamins: all the B vitamins (B1, B2, B3, B5, B6, B12, Folate, Biotin, Choline), and vitamin C.

### Fat-Soluble Vitamins

*Vitamin A*

Vitamin A is actually a complex group of nutrients: retinoids and carotenoids. These nutrients are best known for their importance in eye health but are also critical to proper growth and development, immune function and the health and vitality of the skin. Vitamin A is important to reproduction; manufacture of adrenal and thyroid hormones. It is also essential to proper immune function and supports the function and maintenance of nerve cells.

Juicing Ingredients with high values of vitamin A include:

- Sweet Potato
- Carrots
- Collard Greens
- Kale
- Spinach
- Parsley

*Vitamin D*

Vitamin D is considered by some researchers to be more of a hormone than a vitamin as it is manufactured by the body in response to exposure to sunlight on the skin. It is essential to the absorption of calcium and healthy bones and teeth. Because vitamin D is manufactured in the body it is not a vitamin which is found in fruits and vegetables. It is found in high amounts in cod liver oil, fish, eggs and organ meats.

*Vitamin E*

Vitamin E acts primarily as an antioxidant providing protection to the cells of the body against oxidation. Diets high in vitamin E have been shown to protect against heart disease, stroke, cancer and other degenerative diseases. While the highest sources of vitamin E are found in whole grains and seeds (as it is an oil based vitamin) it is also present in high values in some fruits and vegetables.

Juicing ingredients with high values of vitamin E include:
- Wheatgrass/Barley Grass/Oat Grass
- Spinach
- Swiss Chard
- Turnip Greens

*Vitamin K*

Vitamin K is found in green leafy vegetables (K1) and is also synthesized in the body (K3). It is critical to bone health and bone growth, and is important in the mineralization of bones. Deficiencies lead to poor mineralization of bones which can result in susceptibility to bone injury and breaks of bones being more severe and difficult to heal. K1 is superior in this mineralization to K3 and thus the dietary requirement for vitamin K.

- Kale
- Turnip Greens
- Spinach
- Broccoli
- Lettuce
- Cabbage

## Water-Soluble Vitamins

*B Vitamins*

The B vitamins can be confusing because they often go by other names. Here is a table to make it simple:

| | |
|---|---|
| **Vitamin B1** | Thiamine |
| **Vitamin B2** | Riboflavin |
| **Vitamin B3** | Niacin |
| **Vitamin B5** | Pantothenic Acid |
| **Vitamin B6** | Pyrodoxine |
| **Folate** | Vitamin B9, Methylfolate |
| **Biotin** | Vitamin B7, Coenzyme R, or Vitamin H |
| **Choline** | B vitamin related molecule, produced by the body |
| **Vitamin B12** | Cobolomin |

Folate, Biotin, and Choline are all considered "members of the B vitamin family", as they are key components in how the B vitamins work in the body, and also have other names in the nutritional sciences, which are shown in the chart but are much less commonly called by B vitamin names.

*Vitamin B1 (Thiamine)*

Vitamin B1 is crucial to enzyme function and the metabolizing of carbohydrates. It is also critical to nerve cell function. Vitamin B1 deficiency is relatively uncommon.

Foods containing the highest sources of vitamin B1 are tuna, black beans, sunflower seeds, navy beans, pinto beans, sesame seeds and other members of the bean, pea and seed groups.

*Vitamin B2 (Riboflavin)*

Vitamin B2 is critical to energy production and metabolism. It is critical to the function of two key enzymes in the energy production system. Deficiencies result in decreased energy in cells, particularly replicating cells. Early symptoms of B2 deficiencies include cracking of the lips, and skin in the corners of the mouth, visual disturbances and loss of visual acuity as well as dryness and itching of the eyes.

Juicing ingredients with a high value of vitamin B2 include:

- Spinach
- Collard Greens
- Asparagus
- Zucchini
- Swish Chard
- Broccoli
- Turnip Greens
- Mustard Greens

### Vitamin B3 (Niacin)

Vitamin B3 is another compound that is produced in the body, as well as being available in foods. Vitamin B3 is produced in the body using tryptophan, which is often considered the important nutrient rather than niacin (B3). This is another of the compounds responsible for energy production in the body and is involved in over 50 different chemical processes in the body including the production of adrenal and sex hormones. It helps to control blood sugar levels, lower cholesterol and supports replication and DNA functions in the cells. In its complete form, niacin is most plentiful in poultry, fish (especially tuna and halibut), venison and lamb.

Niacin is available in certain greens and vegetables, but in most cases the levels of tryptophan in those foods is significantly higher than the niacin, and since the body converts the tryptophan to niacin, it makes more sense to look to tryptophan for the nutrient value in juicing ingredients.

Juicing ingredients with a high level of tryptophan include:

- Wheatgrass/Barley Grass/Oat Grass
- Collard Greens
- Swiss Chard
- Turnip Greens
- Mustard Greens
- Spinach
- Kale
- Celery

## Vitamin B5 (Pantothenic Acid)

Vitamin B5 is another important component of energy production in the body, it helps your body convert fats and carbohydrates into energy. It is critical in the production of adrenal hormone and red blood cells. Long known as the 'anti-stress' vitamin, because it is essential to adrenal function and metabolism in cells. Pantothenic acid helps cells with healthy fat production.

Juicing ingredients with high values of vitamin B5 include:
- Wheatgrass/Barley Grass/Oat Grass
- Sweet Potato
- Broccoli
- Collard Greens
- Turnip Greens
- Swiss Chard

## Vitamin B6 (Pyrodoxine)

Vitamin B6 supports nervous system function, the breakdown of sugars and carbohydrates in the body and control of the levels of homocysteine which if not kept in check can build up and lead to cardiovascular disease and heart attack. Vitamin B6 levels in the body seem to be linked to magnesium levels in the body, so food sources high in magnesium are important to vitamin B6 function.

Highest sources come from foods such as brewer's yeast, sunflower seeds, various nuts and beans, bananas and avocados.

Juicing ingredients with high levels of vitamin B6 include:

- Spinach
- Kale
- Sweet Peppers
- Broccoli
- Brussels Sprouts
- Swiss Chard
- Cantaloupe
- Cabbage
- Carrots

*Folate*

Folate is essential to DNA synthesis and every aspect of cell division and replication. This is one reason it is an important nutrient during pregnancy. It is essential in the production of blood cells, muscle, healing and wound repair. It also regulates and reduces levels of homocysteine in the blood, which provides protection against heart disease, stroke and osteoporosis and is essential to the functioning of vitamin B12 in the body.

Most people are deficient in folate, and so the supplement folic acid, a synthetic form of folate, is commonly prescribed. However, there are detrimental impacts to consumption of the synthetic form, and it is far healthier to obtain folate from fruits and vegetables in its natural form. Juicing allows you to increase your daily intake of folate with little effort.

Juicing ingredients with high levels of folate include:

- Wheatgrass/Barley Grass/Oat Grass
- Parsley
- Spinach

- Collard Greens
- Turnip Greens

## Biotin

Biotin works synergistically with Vitamins B2, B3, B6, and Vitamin A to maintain healthy skin, nails, and hair, metabolism of carbohydrates, fats and protein and energy production in the body.

Juicing ingredients with high values of biotin include:
- Swiss Chard

## Choline

Choline is related to the B vitamin family and is produced by the body from lecithin foods. It is used in nerve impulse transmission, cell membrane building and the movement of fats between cells. This makes it important to physical stamina and endurance and physical performance. It is also responsible for production of certain brain chemicals which control neurotransmission and memory, and necessary for proper liver function.

Juicing ingredients with high values of choline include:
- Collard Greens
- Swiss Chard

## Vitamin B12

Vitamin B12 supports the development of red blood cells, prevents anemia and helps the cells metabolize proteins, fats and carbohydrates. It is also important in proper nerve cell function. It is only available from animal products, the highest sources being liver and kidney meats, followed by fish, eggs, meats and cheeses. It is needed in only very small amounts and is measured in mcg (micrograms) for daily intake values.

*Vitamin C Ascorbic Acid*

Vitamin C is a major defender against free radicals and a known cancer risk reducer. It is a nutritional antioxidant and plays a major role in the production of stable collagen, which is needed in the formation of cartilage, connective tissue, ligaments and tendons. In this way, you could say vitamin C holds us together. It is also important in the absorption of other nutrients, in particular, iron. Vitamin C supports immune function and nerve transmission substances and hormones.

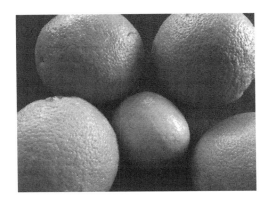

Juicing ingredients with high values of vitamin C include:

- Red bell peppers
- Guavas
- Kale
- Parsley
- Turnip Greens
- Mustard Greens
- Cabbage, Red
- Strawberries
- Papayas
- Spinach
- Oranges
- Kiwi

## Minerals

Minerals are inorganic compounds as they are found in the soil and in deposits beneath the soil, and are not able to be absorbed and assimilated effectively in this form. Otherwise, we would all be fine scooping up and eating handfuls of dirt.

Plants draw up minerals from the soil and store them in their molecular structure, binding them to the plant molecules as they grow. Different types of plant molecular structures bind minerals differently, and in some cases these plant fibers and molecular structures bind the minerals so tightly that it is difficult for us to absorb minerals even from plants.

Juicing fruits and vegetables releases even these tightly bound minerals from the plant fiber, making the minerals much more bio-available to us. This is one of the major benefits of juicing, because the mineral content the juice delivers to your body is higher than it would be if you simply ate the fruit or vegetable in its whole form.

The essential minerals we need for health are classified into two major groups, 'Major' and 'Minor' essential minerals. The classification is not related to their importance as essential minerals. All of these minerals are essential to good health. The classification distinguishes the amount of the minerals required to maintain health. We need 100 milligrams per day of the major essential minerals and less than that of the minor essential minerals.

## Major Essential Minerals
- Calcium
- Phosphorous
- Potassium

- Sodium
- Chloride
- Magnesium

**Minor Essential Minerals (Essential Trace Minerals)**

- Zinc
- Iron
- Manganese
- Copper
- Boron
- Silicon
- Molybdenum
- Vanadium
- Chromium
- Selenium
- Iodine

You will find the minor trace minerals noted in the special notes sections of the *Reference Guide to Great Juicing Ingredients* in the next chapter. Not all of them are listed in the special notes, however a handy online reference guide to find complete nutritional analysis of many foods can be found at WHFoods.com in their main food table of contents. Each food has a full page of information dedicated to it as well as an additional in-depth analysis page which can be found through an individual link in the nutritional profile section of the food's main page.

These in-depth nutritional analysis guides are perhaps the most thorough available online today. The main food table of contents directory is here: http://www.whfoods.com/foodstoc.php.

*Calcium*

Calcium is the most dominant mineral present in the human body. It works in conjunction with phosphorus and magnesium to build bones and teeth. It also stabilizes blood pressure, is essential for blood clotting, communicates information among cells and contributes to normal brain function.

Ratios of calcium to phosphorus and magnesium are critical to good health and for many people calcium and magnesium deficiencies result from diets high in processed foods and low in whole foods. Calcium can also be leached from the body by caffeine, and an over-abundance of phosphorus.

Juicing ingredients with highest calcium levels:
- Collard Greens
- Spinach
- Turnip Greens
- Mustard Greens
- Swiss Chard
- Kale

*Phosphorus*

Phosphorus works with calcium in the body, building strong bones and teeth. It is also essential to cell synthesis, energy production, calcium absorption and metabolism. It is important that the ratios between calcium and phosphorous be balanced. These two minerals work together and provide optimum support in equal amounts. Too much phosphorus will cause the body to leach calcium and eliminate it through the urine. The greater the imbalance (more phosphorus than calcium) the greater the calcium loss will be. Excess phosphorus has been linked to osteoporosis (weakening of bones) which makes sense in this context of calcium loss.

For most of us, getting phosphorus is fairly easy as it is present in most foods, and it is plentiful in things like carbonated beverages. However, calcium is another story and many Americans are deficient in calcium; so it is important to eat foods with balanced calcium/phosphorus levels or even higher calcium than phosphorus levels.

Juicing ingredients with highest values for phosphorus:

- Broccoli
- Brussels Sprouts
- Swiss Chard
- Carrots

Juicing ingredients with ratios of calcium to phosphorus that are higher in calcium:

- Cabbage
- Collard Greens
- Kale
- Mustard Greens
- Parsley

*Magnesium*

Magnesium is an essential mineral which is most predominant in our cells. Second only to potassium in cells, it plays a key role in enzyme activation and in electrical charges and energy exchange. It is critical in the function of calcium and phosphorous as well.

Magnesium deficiency is also a world-wide phenomena; with some international health organizations citing that up to 80 percent of the world's population is magnesium deficient. In the United States it has been presumed that magnesium deficiency is not a critical factor. However, in recent years the increase in processed food consumption and reduction in whole food consumption has dramatically decreased magnesium levels in the typical American diet.

Magnesium deficiency can be a leading factor in heart disease and sudden heart attack and research has demonstrated that many victims of sudden heart attack have had magnesium deficiency in the heart muscle. Magnesium deficiency symptoms can include muscle cramping, numbness and tingling in hands and feet, insomnia and headaches.

Typical RDI numbers for magnesium for adults are around 300mg; however new research suggests that an RDI based on body weight at 6mg per kilogram of body weight may be a more accurate indicator. This would put the 300mg RDI in line with a person weighing 110 pounds.

There are a good number of fresh fruits and vegetables with high magnesium content but they are typically not the most commonly eaten fruits and vegetables in the American diet.

Juicing ingredients with highest magnesium values:

| | |
|---|---|
| Spinach | 156 mg/serving (1 cup) |
| Swiss Chard | 150 mg/serving (1 cup) |
| Collard Greens | 49 mg/ serving (1 cup) |
| Turnip Greens | 31.68 mg/serving (1 cup) |
| Wheat / Barley Grass | 24 mg/serving (100 grams/2.8 ounces) |

*Potassium*

Adequate potassium intake is essential to good health. The typical American diet leads to high sodium levels which negatively impact our potassium levels.

The major culprit in a potassium deficient diet is a lack of fresh fruit and vegetables in the diet and higher consumption of processed foods (containing excessive amounts of various forms of sodium)! So, drink your fruits and veggies and you WILL feel the power. This I can pretty much guarantee. Especially if you are not eating 8 to 10 servings of fruits and vegetables a day when you start juicing. (And who is?)

When you drink a fresh juice and feel instant energy and strength, that is the potassium flooding your system and balancing the potassium/sodium levels in your cells. Because we are all prone to excess sodium in the modern diet, our cells become over-burdened, and our energy drops. Potassium deficiency is a common cause of high blood pressure. It also causes muscle weakness, loss of stored glycogen (energy stores in our body converted from blood sugars for long term energy use), heart irregularities, mental confusion and irritability and nerve function disruptions.

In 2004, the Institute of Medicine at the National Academy of Sciences issued new increased Adequate Intake (AI) levels for potassium. The recommendations are as follows:

| | |
|---|---|
| 0-6 months: | 400 mg |
| 6-12 months: | 700 mg |
| 1-3 years: | 3.5 g |
| 4-8 years: | 3.8 g |
| 9-13 years: | 4.5 g |
| 14-18 years: | 4.5 g |
| 19-30 years: | 4.7 g |
| 31-50 years: | 4.7 g |
| 51+ years: | 4.7 g |
| Pregnant women: | 4.7 g |
| Lactating women: | 5.1 g |

To learn more about advanced research into potassium and its ability to heal the body read any of the books by Charlotte Gerson (see reading recommendations at the end of this book.)

Juicing Ingredients with highest potassium levels include:

| | |
|---|---|
| Swiss Chard | 960 mg/serving (1 cup) |
| Spinach | 838 mg/serving (1 cup) |
| Cantaloupe | 427 mg/serving (1 cup) |
| Tomatoes | 426 mg/serving (1 cup) |
| Carrots | 390 mg/serving (1 cup) |
| Fennel | 360 mg/serving (1 cup) |
| Brussels Sprouts | 342 mg/serving (1 cup) |

## Sodium & Chloride

Recommended dietary intake of potassium to sodium and chloride are 4.7g/ 1.5g/ 2.3g.

Most of us are getting too much sodium and chloride in our modern diets. The relationship between potassium and sodium is a key component to good health.

Recent research suggests the optimum minimum ratio of 5:1 potassium to sodium; however for most Americans the ratio is actually more like 1:2. This imbalance is a serious health issue, and potassium deficiency, even when there is enough potassium in the diet, is the result. The over-abundance of sodium upsets the proper balance of these two essential minerals. As much as 50 percent of excess sodium comes from processed foods. Table salt (sodium chloride) accounts for approximately 5 percent of dietary intake.

The potassium/sodium ratios in fruits and vegetables as they naturally occur are an indicator of what is healthy for us, as most of the sodium we consume comes not from the natural sodium in foods we eat but from salt added during cooking, in food processing and as a condiment (table salt). Additionally many of the salts used in modern food packaging and preparations of packaged foods are toxic to our bodies.

Chloride is present as potassium chloride in many foods, and in many salts. It is through the sodium chlorides that our chloride levels are elevated in the modern diet. Chloride deficiency can occur if major fluid loss through illness occurs, and is a key component in stomach juices and fluid regulation. Otherwise, deficiency is rare.

Here are a few examples of juicing ingredients with excellent potassium/sodium ratios to help improve your potassium/sodium balance:

| | |
|---|---|
| Peaches, Plums | 150-1 |
| Strawberries | 122->1 |
| Tomato | 98-1 |
| Apples | 90:1 |
| Carrots | 75:1 |
| Oranges | 260:1 |

Celery is a juicing ingredient with high values of sodium chloride in their natural form. Celery's potassium/sodium ratio is approximately 3.5-1.


## Vitamins, Minerals and Organic, Conventional or GM Foods

Recent research has revealed that many fruits and vegetables have very specific antioxidant, anti-inflammatory and immune building properties which are higher in organically grown fruits and vegetables than in 'conventionally' grown foods. More long standing research has clearly demonstrated that soil health and particularly healthy microorganism and bacteria life in soils dramatically impacts the ability of plants to take up nutrients, minerals, long chain amino acids, sugars and other key components to healthy plant growth.

In recent years, the 'public debate' over organic versus conventional farming practices and its impact on food quality has largely drowned out the actual scientific data. On top of this, big agriculture sponsored 'research' has 'demonstrated' no difference between organic and conventionally grown food. A great deal of money has gone into 'proving' this case. But the facts are hard to dispute when independent researchers continue to validate the higher levels of minerals, vitamins and phytochemicals in organically grown foods.

A comparative study of corn nutrition between GM and non GM corn crops of 2011 has now begun to gain national attention as it reveals that not only is the mineral content of the GM corn virtually non-existent, but that the GM corn also contains levels of toxins which far exceed EPA and FDA standards for safety. You can find more information at

http://www.naturalnews.com/039864_GMO_corn_nutrients_minerals.html.

As you will see in the *Reference Guide to Great Juicing Ingredients*, new research is emerging which clearly identifies significantly higher values for important nutrition in organic blueberries, organic grapes, and many other organic fruits and vegetables than in their non-organic counterparts.

Based on our own research, and a frustrating inability to get clear information about conventional crops and what chemicals are being used in their production, we have more or less given up on all but a few conventionally grown fruits and vegetables. We still buy conventional oranges and citrus if it is the only citrus available. Otherwise, we simply change out the fruits and vegetables we buy for what *is* available organically grown. It just isn't worth the risk to us any longer.

Just as we've given up all commercially sold meats other than those we can source locally as 100 percent grass fed, free range or pasture raised animals, we've simply eliminated the world of processed foods and conventionally grown produce from our diet.

This may seem somewhat extreme to those who have not done their own research to know how these 'foods' are produced or what the real history of food production over the last 40 or 50 years has been in the United States, but we promise you, we are not radical and we are not extremist. We are very concerned with our health and the health of those we love. Happily, our children have, for the most part, followed or led us in this change of thinking about what we eat.

As a final note, if you have the stomach for it, you may wish to read the bestselling book "*Salt Sugar Fat: How the Food Giants Hooked Us*" by Michael Moss, which exposes the history of food production and marketing in the United States over the past four decades. It is not a pretty picture.

# Reference Guide to Great Juicing Ingredients

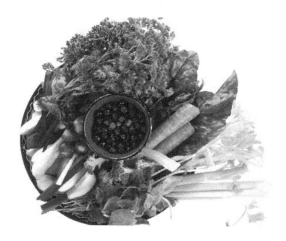

This guide is organized into three main groups:

> ➤ Vegetables
> ➤ Fruits
> ➤ Specialty Herbs

The vegetables are listed by plant family because the health benefits and properties within the plant families are similar. You can mix and match individual members of any of the vegetable families to suit your taste.

Of course, in each vegetable family, some special individual members will have particular health benefits the others may not have, or may not have in as high concentrations. But in general, the vegetable families have similar nutritional benefits within each group.

Fruits are listed after the vegetables, followed by specialty herbs which are not members of the vegetable families.

Recent studies of beets, beet greens and chard have demonstrated this connection within the vegetable family groups.

Characteristics of certain phytonutrients present in the pigment cells of these vegetables have specific beneficial effects on human health. These benefits are specific to the beetroot family of plants and not found in other fruits or vegetables. Tied to the pigment cells of the deep red, yellow, pink, and dark green of leafy chards, the deep red of beets and the deep green of spinach, these phytonutrients provide blood sugar level support, reduce blood pressure and improve vision.

By becoming familiar with the particular traits of each of the vegetable families you can easily select a variety of ingredients for juicing with a full spectrum of health benefits.

There is still a great deal to learn about the powerful micro- and phyto-nutrients in fruits, vegetables and herbs. Ongoing research is uncovering new information every day. One thing is certain, these new studies and their discoveries make it very clear that healthy organic produce provides an important support system for human health in everything from bone strength to illness prevention and much, much more.

Recent research demonstrates that members of the cabbage family fight cancer and help restore our immune function. The latest research on the beetroot family makes it clear that beets, chard and spinach can protect our hearts and vascular system.

There is no easier or simpler way to increase our consumption of these health giving foods than by juicing, and it's very simple to work out a balanced blend of the greens (which can be very astringent, or 'sharp' tasting), and the milder, sweeter fruits and vegetables.

When using beets, carrots or sweet potatoes in the juice, you may not find it necessary to include apple, or other fruits to lighten or sweeten the juice, as these vegetables will provide all the sweetness you need to counter even the strongest of greens.

On the other hand, there are serious benefits to adding green apples, pears and other fruits, (particularly berries) to your diet as regularly as possible. You'll find lots of exciting new information in the sections for each of these individual produce choices in this guide.

In general, try to experiment a little each week, adding or adjusting the ingredients you include in any one juicing session. By adding herbs like mint, basil, parsley, cilantro, ginger or turmeric you can also dramatically increase the health value of the juice and have fun playing with the taste at the same time.

The world of advanced nutrition is actually a fairly new field of science and there is a great deal yet to be discovered. However, there is one trend that seems to be emerging across the research and that is the idea of whole foods. In study after study the benefits of consuming whole natural foods with all their complex phytonutrients, peptides, enzymatic make-up and interconnected nutritional components perform better at providing increased health benefits than individual components of the same foods separated out and consumed alone.

A great example of this is the root turmeric and one of its phytochemicals, curcumin. Curcumin has been shown in many studies to be effective at blocking the formation of beta-amyloid, the substance which causes the formation of plaque and slowing of cerebral function in Alzheimer's disease.

Further advanced study has proven that there are actually several other phytochemicals contained in Turmeric which also are very effective in this same action of blocking beta-amyloid formation, and that indeed, whole turmeric root extracts are more potent and powerful than extracts only containing curcumin in preventing Alzheimer's and Glaucoma, two diseases Turmeric is now known to help prevent.

Just another indication that whole foods and whole fresh juices extracted from whole foods are a super-efficient way to add nutritional value to your diet.

Here are the plant groups and the members of the group suitable for juicing along with a general list of their health benefits and special notes on specific benefits currently known.

## Vegetables

### Asteracea/Daisy Family

- Dandelion
- Endive/Escarole
- Lettuce
- Sunflower*

In general, good sources of vitamins A, K and C, manganese, potassium, calcium and iron.

*Health Benefits:*
Supportive of healthy digestion and metabolism function, these foods also provide good cholesterol and blood sugar regulation. Anti-inflammatory and detoxifying to the digestive tract.

*Special Notes:*
Romaine Lettuce is a highly nutrient-dense lettuce and is preferred. Excellent source of vitamins A, K and C as well as folate. Very good source of manganese, potassium and iron. Good source of vitamin B1, B2, B6, Omega-3 fats, magnesium, calcium, phosphorus, copper, and molybdenum. Cholesterol lowering and heart healthy.

Green and red leaf, butter and specialty lettuce are also now getting more attention in health research. Look for brightness of color, firmness and strength of leaves.

Dandelion greens are another strong green, with many health benefits including supporting kidney function, digestion, circulation and skin health. Great source of calcium, iron, magnesium, potassium and vitamin A. As with most of the super potent greens, a little goes a long way; use small leaves and sparingly, mixing with fruit, carrot and other juices to taste.

Endive is an excellent source of beta-carotene and vitamins B and C, calcium, iron, magnesium, and zinc. Also a very good source of folate and selenium. Endive is a potent green. Use small leaves and in moderation!

*Sunflower is obviously not something you can juice; however you can make exceptional sunflower butter with raw hulled sunflower seeds using your Omega juicer and the blank cone insert. Sunflower seeds are extremely nutritious and delicious.


## Chenopodiaceae/Beetroot Family

- Beet (roots and greens)
- Swiss Chard
- Spinach

In general, excellent sources of Vitamin K, Vitamin A, iron, magnesium, Folate, manganese, Vitamin C, potassium and Vitamin E.

*Health Benefits:*

Anti-inflammatory, antioxidant, support detoxification, vascular and heart health.

The Chenopod family of foods has shown special properties of phytonutrients not found in other foods. Their actions include helping to regulate blood sugar levels and increasing heart and vascular health.

Recent research involving the betacyanine pigments has demonstrated important antioxidant, anti-inflammatory and detoxification support which operate in specialized ways still being researched and are not yet fully understood.

*Special Notes:*

Beets have just been shown to reduce the risk of heart attack by up to fifty percent if taken in a raw juice form in quantities as small as 100 grams a day. Laboratory research has also demonstrated that the antioxidant and anti-inflammatory molecules in beets have the potential to be extremely cancer preventive. Beet greens are also an especially good source of lutein, which research has demonstrated is an important eye health support nutrient and aids in prevention of glaucoma and age related macular degeneration. Excellent source of folate, very good source of manganese, potassium, vitamin C. Good source of magnesium, iron, phosphorus, and copper.

Swiss Chard contains multiple types of betacyanine pigments (not just the dark red/purples but also the yellows and greens) which, in combination offer additional nutritive support in detoxification and blood sugar level control. Excellent source of vitamins K, A, and C, magnesium, manganese, potassium, iron, and vitamin E. Very good source of copper, choline, calcium, vitamin B2, vitamin B6, tryptophan, and protein. Good source of phosphorus, vitamin B1, folate, zinc, biotin, vitamin B3 and vitamin B5.

Spinach is another one of the super producers when it comes to high levels of nutrition. It is rated as an excellent high source for all of the following: Vitamin K, vitamin A, manganese, folate, magnesium, iron, vitamin C, vitamin B2, calcium, potassium, vitamin B6 and vitamin E. Very good source of copper, vitamin B1, protein, phosphorus, zinc, and choline. Good source of Omega-3 fats, vitamin B3, selenium, and tryptophan.

## Convolvulaceae/Sweet Potato Family

- Sweet Potatoes

Excellent source of vitamin A. Very good source of vitamin C and manganese, good source of vitamin B6, potassium, vitamin B5, copper, and vitamin B3.

*Health Benefits:*
Health Benefits of sweet potatoes include specialized antioxidant properties which are related to their sporamins content, a substance the sweet potato uses to repair any damage to its own skin. Sweet potatoes provide excellent beta-carotene support and can be important in removing heavy metals from the digestive tract. You can improve beta-carotene intake from sweet potatoes by adding a small amount of olive oil.

*Special Notes:*
In the United States two different types of sweet potato are sold. One is hard and generally has a light to yellow colored flesh and pale tan skin. The other is soft and generally has a pink to dark red skin and bright orange flesh. The soft varieties (e.g. Jewel and Georgia Jet) are commonly sold as yams in local markets. However, they are not true yams, they are sweet potatoes. This is good to know when determining the nutritive value of your juicing ingredients. Happily, sweet potatoes tend to have higher nutritional content than yams.

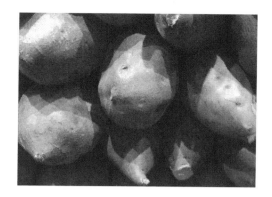

## Crucifer/Cabbage/Mustard Family

- Bok Choy
- Broccoli
- Broccoli Raab
- Brussels Sprouts
- Cabbage
- Cauliflower
- Chinese Cabbage
- Collard Greens
- Cress (Garden or Land Cress)
- Kale
- Kohlrabi
- Mustard Greens
- Radish
- Daikon Radish
- Horse Radish
- Rutabaga
- Turnip
- Watercress

In general excellent sources of vitamin K and vitamin C, and folate. Also a very good source of vitamin A, calcium, manganese, magnesium, potassium, phosphorous, molybdenum, tryptophan, various B vitamins, (proportions alter slightly throughout the group), iron, selenium and Choline.

*Health Benefits:*
Cholesterol reduction (best when steamed, but also present when raw or juiced), anti-inflammatory, antioxidant, detoxifying, cancer-preventive.

*Special Notes:*
Broccoli: Excellent source of vitamin C, K and folate. Very good source of vitamin A, manganese, potassium, vitamin B6, B2, phosphorus, and molybdenum. Good source of vitamin B5, protein, magnesium, calcium, choline, vitamin B1, selenium, and vitamin B3.

Brussels Sprouts: Excellent source of vitamin K and C, very good source of manganese and folate, vitamin A, potassium, vitamin B6 and B1, and molybdenum. Good source of iron, phosphorus, protein, magnesium, vitamin B2, choline, vitamin E, Omega-3 fats, calcium, and vitamin B3.

Cabbage: Excellent source of vitamins K and C. Very good source of folate, manganese, and molybdenum. Good source of vitamin B6, potassium, calcium, and vitamin B1. Cabbage, surprisingly, is also high in Omega 3 Fatty Acids (the same fatty acids found in Salmon and Flax Seed).

Collard Greens: Excellent source of vitamins K, A, and C, folate, manganese, calcium. Very good source of choline, iron, vitamins B6 and B2, magnesium, and tryptophan. Good sources of vitamin E, protein, Omega-3 fats, potassium, phosphorus, vitamins

B1, B3, B5. Collard greens have recently been shown to have an even higher cholesterol lowering effect than any of the other cruciferous foods. Their ability to bind bile acids (which are made of cholesterol) and carry them through the digestive tract to excretion is unsurpassed even by kale. In addition, collard greens have special cancer-preventive properties thanks to their phytonutrient glucosinolates. These agents provide specialized detoxifying and anti-inflammatory support.

Broccoli, cabbage and Brussels sprouts are all very high in vitamins C and K as well as folate and manganese.

Kale is a superstar in vitamins C, A and K and also high in manganese and in copper, which is important in maintaining healthy bones. It is also at the top of the charts for vitamin B6, calcium and potassium. Kale is also a good source of iron, magnesium, vitamin E, Omega-3 fats, vitamin B1, B2 and B3, protein, folate, phosphorus, and tryptophan.

Mustard Greens are excellent sources of vitamins K, A, and C, folate, manganese, and calcium. They are very good sources of vitamins E and B6, potassium, protein, copper, iron, phosphorus, magnesium, and tryptophan.

Turnip greens, like collard greens are also rich in cancer fighting glucosinolates and offer excellent cancer-preventive support. They are also super high in calcium, higher than any other of the cruciferous foods. Excellent sources of vitamins A, C, E and K, as well as copper, manganese, folate, and calcium. They are very good sources of potassium, magnesium, iron, vitamin B2, and tryptophan. Good source of B vitamins and Omega-3 fats.

Unfortunately, in many shops, the greens are removed from the turnips before they are put out for sale. You may have better luck at a farmers market; although often there too the greens are removed when the turnips are harvested. Put in a request to the farmers you buy from to let them know you'd like to buy the greens as well.

While turnips themselves are an excellent food and great juicing material, the leaves have such intensely beneficial properties it is well worth it to make turnip greens a regular part of your diet and juicing regimen.

Another way to ensure a good supply of turnip greens is to grow them yourself. They are extremely hardy and easy to grow, and there are many heirloom turnip seed varieties which can be grown and harvested for seed to maintain an ongoing supply. They are cool weather crops, doing best in spring and fall. Harvest the leaves when they are young, before the turnips are mature and before flowering. The larger and older they are the tougher and more bitter they become. Bitterness is a marker for high calcium content in leafy green vegetables.


## Cucurbit/Squash Family

- Cucumber
- Pumpkin
- Zucchini

In general, good sources of vitamins A, C and B6, manganese and potassium. Specialized carotenoids, alpha and beta-carotenes as well as lutein. Good sources of polysaccharides which protect against diabetes.

*Health Benefits:*

Antioxidant and anti-inflammatory. In particular, all members of this family contain cucurbitacins which provide specific anti-cancer protection against cancers such as uterine, breast and prostate.

Cucumbers are an especially good source of the cucurbitacins for which this food family is known; fresh cucumber phytonutrients, particularly the flavonoids and lignans provide exceptional good antioxidant, anti-inflammatory and anti-cancer protection. Excellent source of vitamin K, and good source of vitamins B5 and C, potassium, magnesium, manganese, and molybdenum.

Pumpkins provide an excellent source of vitamins A and C, and are very good sources of vitamin B6 and manganese. They are also good sources for vitamin K, vitamin B2, potassium, folate, copper, Omega-3 fats and magnesium.

Zucchini has recently been found to contain some important anti-cancer properties with some phytonutrient components having demonstrated the ability to block certain cancer growth pathways. It is an excellent source of vitamins C and B6, as well as manganese. It is a very good source of vitamin B2, potassium and folate. Zucchini is also a good source of magnesium, vitamins A, K, B1, and B3, phosphorus, copper, molybdenum, and Omega-3 fats.

## Dioscorea/Yam Family

- Yams

In general, good source of vitamins C and B6, potassium, manganese, and phytoestrogens.

*Health Benefits:*
Yams provide support for cardio-vascular health, and are a good source of vitamins C and B6, as well as potassium and manganese. They contain diosgenin and have phytoestrogen properties which

support healthy hormone function. It is their high level of vitamin B6 which aids in the detoxification of excess estrogen.

*Special Notes:*

Please note, as mentioned earlier in the book, the vast majority of vegetables sold as yams in the United States are actually orange fleshed sweet potatoes. We have even interviewed produce specialists in local markets who tell us they do not, and have not ever, carried true yams in their markets. We include them here for those outside the US who may, in fact, have access to true yams.

## Fabaceae/Bean/Pea Family

We really don't juice any of the foods in this family, although I suppose we could juice alfalfa or alfalfa greens. Most of the members of this family are wonderfully good for you, including green beans, adzuki beans, chickpeas and others, but they do not make for good juicing material.

## Solanaceae/Nightshade/Potato Family

- Bell peppers
- Tomato
- Tomatillo

Also in this family, although not widely cultivated or researched as yet are:

- Ground Cherry
- Goose Berry/Wolf Berry

Note: Nightshades are a group of plants to which some people are very sensitive. If you cannot tolerate tomatoes, potatoes or peppers, it is best not to juice them either.

In general, excellent source of vitamins C, A, E, K and B6 as well as folate. This family is known for high levels of lycopenes. In fact, bell peppers and tomatoes are the only two plant foods which contain over two thirds of the full range of carotenoids found in fruits and vegetables.

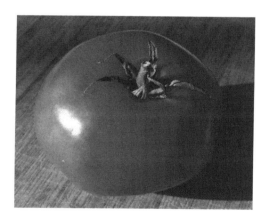

*Health Benefits:*
Health Benefits include the properties of the lycopenes which are known for their antioxidant protection and support of bone health.

*Special Notes:*
Bell Peppers are also a good source of vitamins B1, B2, and B3, potassium, magnesium, manganese, and molybdenum.

Tomatoes are also good sources of copper, vitamin E, phosphorus, and protein.

## Poaceae/Grasses Family

- Barley Grass
- Wheat Grass
- Oat Grass

Excellent source of chlorophyll, as well as a complete amino acid profile. Also excellent source of vitamins A, C and B2, calcium, iron, a very broad spectrum of trace minerals, and tryptophan.

*Health benefits:*

These three members of the grass family are the standout superstars of their family. High in chlorophyll, all of the eight essential amino acids and jam-packed with minerals, they are not only extremely nutrient dense, they are superbly bio-available. That means that as soon as you drink juice made with them it goes right to work throughout your body.

They have more vitamin C than oranges and more iron than spinach; all three are higher in calcium than milk and have high levels of vitamin B1.

The high levels of chlorophyll in these grasses give them additional benefit to your body in several ways. First, the chlorophyll delivers oxygen directly to your cells. It is also nearly identical to the hemoglobin in your blood and so it supports and cleanses both the blood and the liver.

The grasses are liver cleansing and boost digestive acids in the stomach. Due to acid reflux and other symptoms, many people erroneously assume their stomach is too acidic. Research has shown the exact opposite to be true. Lower levels of hydrochloric acid in the stomach can result in symptoms such as acid reflux. These grasses also help our bodies to eliminate toxic heavy metals, and contain the complete spectrum of the eight essential amino acids our bodies cannot produce on their own. This means that grass juices can break down the proteins our bodies need. Extreme bio-availability also means they can help in the body's elimination of stored toxins in the colon.

*Special Notes:*

The complete amino acid profile and trace mineral content of these grasses make them a true superfood for the blood and vital organs of the body. In fact, you will find many sources for these superfoods as a dry green powder sold by nutritional supplement companies. This is one way to get their benefit into your juice.

The alternative is to grow your own. It is super-fast, super-easy and relatively inexpensive to do. When compared to the cost of dry powders, it is far less costly.

Should you choose to grow your own barley grass, oat grass, or wheatgrass you can also add a small amount of Azomite trace mineral powder to the soil mix - a very light top dressing is all you need. This will seriously boost the trace mineral content of your grasses.

> ➡ TIP: Source for Grass Seeds, Grass Seed Kits, and Azomite: http://www.wheatgrasskits.com

We've been growing our own barley grass for a couple of years now. It produces huge abundant crops quickly and easily (I think it might be the easiest thing on earth to grow) and it grows FAST. I've included a series of photos here to show you the time it takes to go from a box of seeds placed on top of nice compost and soil mix with Azomite to six to eight inch tall bushy greens ready for cutting and juicing.

Day 1 - Barley Grass Seeds spread on top of soil and watered in:

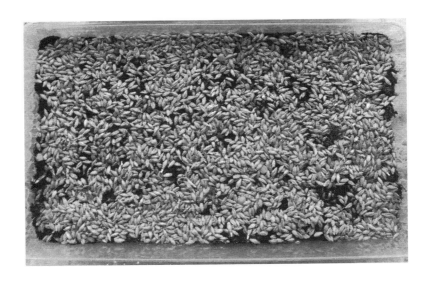

Days 2 to 4 – Seeds are watered daily so they stay moist. We also mist them with a spray bottle (once a day is fine.)

Day 5 – Barley grass seeds have begun to sprout:

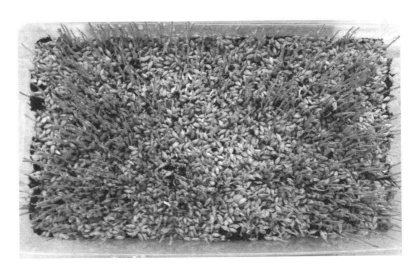

Day 6 – Most seeds have sprouted and the grass is about 2 inches tall:

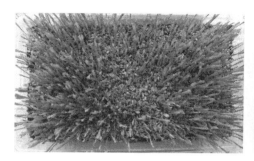 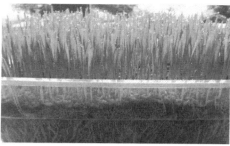

Day 7 – Grass is getting longer fast, and also darker in color:

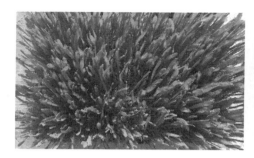 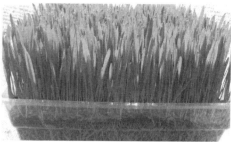

Day 8 - Almost ready for juicing:

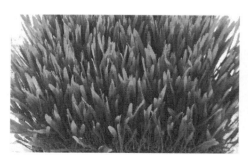 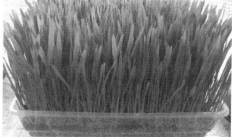

Day 9 – We're there! Cut the grass with scissors leaving about half an inch to an inch so it can regrow one more time. Juice the cut grass immediately:

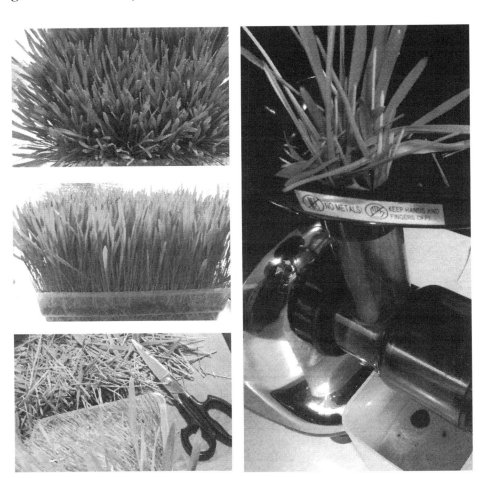

One word of caution about barley grass: it is very good for you and extremely high in all the good nutrients bright greens offer, but it is extremely sharp and green tasting. If you are not used to green juices, you will definitely want to temper it with lemon, apple, beet, carrot or sweet potato to mellow out the taste. The first time I had a straight up barley grass juice I nearly spit it across the room my mouth was so shocked by the intensity of it! So, add *small* amounts to your mixed veggie and fruit juices to start, until you develop a taste for it.

## Umbelliferae/Carrot Family

- Carrot
- Celery
- Celeriac
- Chervil
- Coriander/Cilantro
- Dill
- Fennel
- Parsley
- Parsnip
- Root parsley

In general, good sources of vitamins A, K, C and B6.

*Health Benefits:*

Antioxidant, cardiovascular health promoter, anti-cancer benefits - particularly colon cancer, eye/vision health (most well known in association with its high concentration of vitamin A)

*Special Notes:*

Carrots: Most well known as an excellent source of beta-carotene (vitamin A), carrots are also excellent in preventing cancer (particularly colon cancer) as European studies have shown. Carrots are also a very good source of vitamins K and C, and potassium, and a good source of manganese, molybdenum, all the B vitamins, vitamin E, folate, and phosphorus.

Celery is another less well known super defender. Research has shown its special class of phytonutrients can prevent inflammatory response in the digestive tract, reduce tumor activity and protect body fats and blood vessel walls from oxidative damage. Look for more news on celery with new emerging research but don't wait to incorporate it into your daily juicing regimen. Celery is an excellent source of vitamin K, as well as a very good source of vitamins A and C, folate, potassium, manganese, and molybdenum. Celery provides a good source of vitamins B2 and B5, calcium, magnesium, and tryptophan.

Cilantro (and its dry seed form coriander) is known in some parts of the world as an anti-diabetic herb. It has been proven to stimulate the secretion of insulin in diabetic mice and lower blood sugar. It has also demonstrated the ability to lower cholesterol and the production of free radicals in the body. Its broad spectrum of phytonutrients gives it a distinguished place among the healing herbs.

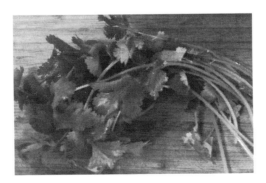

Cilantro is a very good source of vitamins A, C, E, K, B2, B3, B5, and B6 and folate. It's a good source of calcium, iron, magnesium, manganese, phosphorus, potassium and copper.

Surprisingly, cilantro has also recently been proven to contain what may be the strongest antibiotic agent found in live plants. Its capacity to kill salmonella was demonstrated to be twice as powerful as the leading pharmaceutical antibiotic. It is abundantly available in most areas year round, so by adding it to your juicing regimen you can achieve protection against food poisoning as well as regulating blood sugar, lowering cholesterol and flooding your body with health enhancing phytonutrients.

Parsley is classified as a 'chemoprotective' food as its volatile oils actually help the body defend against molecular degradation due to oxidation and specific carcinogens. It is also an important defender against rheumatoid arthritis. Parsley is an excellent source of vitamins K, C, and A. Parsley is also a good source of iron and folate. (Remember to mix it with citrus to get the best iron absorption and increase the levels of calcium you can absorb from the citrus as well.)

Parsnips, like carrots are a root vegetable, sweet in flavor. Unlike carrots they are not a source of beta-carotene, but are instead very high in Folate as well as having the same cholesterol lowering and blood sugar regulating properties as carrots.

Dill, like parsley, is another of the 'chemoprotective' foods, which can help neutralize certain carcinogens. Dill is also bacteriostatic, like garlic; regulating bacteria growth in the body. Dill also protects against bone loss through its mineral content. It is a very good source of calcium, and a good source of manganese, iron, and magnesium.

Fennel is another special phytonutrient producer with a volatile oil which has been shown to be effective against cancer, protect against oxidation and reduce inflammatory response in cells. It has the added benefit of being in season in winter and early spring when many other vegetables are not available. Fennel is an excellent source of vitamin C and a very good source of potassium, manganese, and folate. It's a good source of phosphorus, calcium, magnesium, iron and copper, and molybdenum.

**Fruits**

**Apples**

Good source of vitamin C.

*Health Benefits:*

Apples can help control blood sugar in multiple ways due to their apple polyphenols. Apples have been shown to reduce blood fat content. Apples also have the potential to balance bacteria in the digestive tract. Recent studies have demonstrated that the phytonutrients in apples play an important role in digestive health.

> ➡ TIP: When selecting Apples for juicing lean toward green, firm and crisp. Mealy, overripe and dark red apples tend to make more mush and foam in the juicer.

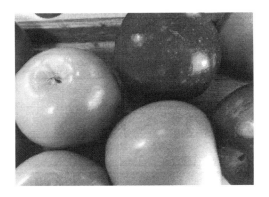

**Blueberries**

Excellent source of vitamin K and a very good source of vitamin C and manganese.

*Health Benefits:*

Blueberries have high antioxidant properties as well as being shown to have an important ability to regulate blood sugar in type 2 diabetic patients. Recent studies have demonstrated that a blueberry juice made up of 3/4 of a pound of blueberries (yields one cup of juice) caused measurable and significant improvement in memory function in the elderly. Another study clearly demonstrated that organic blueberries had significantly higher antioxidant properties than conventionally grown blueberries, so it is important to buy organic blueberries.

## Cantaloupe

Cantaloupe is a power house in the fruits category containing high nutritional value typical for the cucurbit family of which all melons are members. It is an excellent source of vitamins A and C and a very good source of potassium as well as a good source of B vitamins 1, 3, and 6, vitamin K, folate, and magnesium. One cup contains over 100% of the recommended daily intake of vitamin A.

*Health Benefits:*

High beta-carotene content and low glycemic index. Benefits include support to vision health, blood sugar regulation and general reduction of inflammation in the body.

## Cranberries

Excellent source of vitamin C, and a good source of vitamins E and K as well as manganese and a multitude of phytonutrients.

*Health benefits:*

Anti-inflammatory, antioxidant, and anti-cancer properties. Cranberry has long been used to treat urinary tract infections, and new research has identified exactly how the cranberry accomplishes this through some of its specialized phytonutrients. Cranberry also reduces risk for periodontal and heart disease.

**Grapefruit**

Excellent source of vitamins C and A, lycopene (in pink and yellow grapefruit) and liminoids. Good source of vitamins B1, B5, and potassium.

*Health Benefits:*

All vitamin C rich fruits and vegetables help ward off colds and flu. A recent Asian study has shown that the lycopenes in grapefruit, highest in pink and not present in white grapefruit, have been proven to be important in reducing the risk of prostate cancer. Liminoids, proven as effective cancer fighters, are also present in grapefruit. New studies demonstrate grapefruit may also be effective in lowering cholesterol in humans. Long term research has shown grapefruit juice to be useful in preventing kidney stones as well.

**Grapes**

Excellent source of manganese, very good source of vitamin K, and good source of vitamins C, B1, and B6, and potassium. Grapes contain vital phytonutrients including resveratrol.

*Health Benefits:*

Grapes have low glycemic value and balance blood sugar. Resveratrol has also been linked to longevity through induction of the expression of certain longevity genes.

> ➡ TIP: Grapes have a definite proven record of being high in pesticide residues in the table grape or 'grapes for eating' varieties. Only use organically grown grapes in juicing.

## Kiwi

Excellent source of vitamin C, as well as a good source of potassium and beneficial phytonutrients. One serving of Kiwi (one fruit) contains 120% of the Recommended Dietary Allowance for vitamin C. High levels of antioxidant carotenoids and flavonoids are contained as well.

*Health benefits:*

The phytonutrients in kiwi protect DNA in human cells, as demonstrated in Italian studies, although the active agent responsible for this is still undetermined. Protects against arthritis, rheumatoid arthritis, asthma and respiratory infections. Also effective in protecting against certain cancers, and supporting cardiovascular health.

## Lemons & Limes

Excellent source of Vitamin C, bioflavonoids, and phytonutrients.

*Health benefits:*

Same range of benefits from all high vitamin C fruits and vegetables, including strong antioxidant powers, rich source of limonin and other essential nutrients which aid the body in defending against cancers, arthritis and certain diseases.

While not as powerful a source of Vitamin C as kiwi, lemons and limes have the added benefit of working very well to brighten and balance strong green juices, making them an excellent source of the benefits of citrus to add to any juice recipe. In addition they contain the limonin, bioflavonoids, and essential nutrients which support good health.

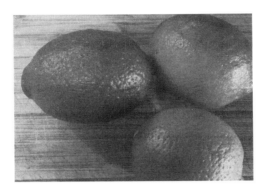

**Nectarines**

Very good source of vitamin C, lutein, and lycopene. Good source of vitamin A, potassium, and niacin.

*Health benefits:*

Antioxidant and anti-tumor properties, protect against heart disease, reduce the risk of cancer and macular degeneration.

**Pears**

Very good source of vitamins C and K. Special class of flavonoids, antioxidants.

*Health benefits:*
Significant protection against type 2 diabetes. The skins of pears contain up to 40% of the flavonoids providing this protection.

➡ TIP: A combination of apples and pears was found to be most effective and red skinned pears have all three of the most important phytonutrients important to the protection from diabetes. By combining pears and apples together in juices you provide your body with all the important bioflavonoids needed to protect and support optimal health.

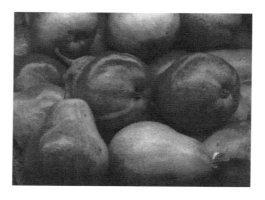

**Peaches**

Very good source of vitamin C, Lutein, and Lycopene. Good source of vitamin A, potassium, and niacin.

*Health benefits:*

Antioxidant and anti-tumor properties, protect against heart disease, reduce the risk of cancer and macular degeneration.

## Pineapple

Excellent source of vitamin C and manganese and a good source of vitamins B1 and B6 as well as copper and folate.

*Health benefits:*

All benefits associated with vitamin C as well as increased energy and cell support due to the high levels of manganese. Anecdotal evidence suggests pineapple is a good digestive aid, although the particular role of the bromelains it contains is still under research. It does seem to suggest that certain components of bromelain assist in digestion and digestive tract health.

## Plums

Very good source of vitamin C. Plums are also a good source of vitamins A and K and potassium.

*Health Benefits:*

Plums are a very good source of vitamin C and provide support for the uptake of iron and increase the antioxidant protection provided by vitamin C. Plums are high in phenolic compounds which are known to strengthen the immune system.

**Raspberries**

Excellent source of vitamin C and manganese. Raspberries, like all berries, are nutritionally dense. They are a very good source of vitamin K and a good source of magnesium, folate, copper, Omega-3 fats, potassium, and vitamin E.

*Health Benefits:*
These berries, like blueberries have powerful antioxidant and anti-inflammatory properties. Also like blueberries, recent studies have shown that organic raspberries are significantly higher in their antioxidant and anti-inflammatory properties than conventionally grown fruits. So buy organic.

Finally, new research indicates that certain phytonutrients in raspberries are capable of increasing the burn rates within our cells (speeding up metabolism) as well as blocking certain fat digestion processes. Research is underway to determine if these raspberry ketones may be effective in weight management.

**Strawberries**

Excellent source of Vitamin C and manganese, as well as a very good source of folate and iodine. Strawberries are a good source of potassium, magnesium, Omega-3 fats, and vitamin K.

*Health Benefits:*
Strawberries, blackberries and cranberries are at the top of the antioxidant fruit category, with blackberries being highest while strawberries are in the #4 position. However, in most circumstances, people tend to consume a larger quantity of strawberries than blackberries, especially in their raw whole fruit

form, so they can actually end up being the highest source of antioxidant fruit consumed; particularly in America.

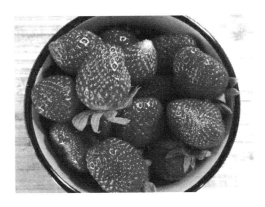

> ➡ TIP: Strawberries have an additional power that has only recently been discovered: when eaten at the same time as table sugar they have the power to counteract the blood sugar/insulin spike that normally occurs when eating white sugar. Strawberries are very fragile and lose their nutrient value quickly - usually within 3 days. Keep them extra chilled and contained in the fridge to prevent the air circulation in the fridge from further reducing their nutrition value.

**Watermelons**

Excellent source of vitamin C and a very good source of vitamin A. High in lycopene and citrulline, important cardiovascular health supporting phytonutrients. They are also good sources of potassium and magnesium.

*Health Benefits:*

Recent research has revealed that watermelons are exceptional sources of lycopene, an important phytonutrient for heart health. Watermelons and tomatoes have high concentrations of lycopene, as do pink grapefruits. Another important phytonutrient getting attention in research is citrulline, which also contributes to heart health, circulation and may even help in the body's regulation of the accumulation of fat in fat cells.

## Specialty Herbs

Each of the following herbs contain volatile oils and special compounds which distinguish them from other food plants and which are now being found to contain an extensive array of healing properties due to unique chemical compounds and components within them. While some of these plants offer similar health benefits, they each have their own special flavors and properties. Whether the warming energy of cinnamon or the soothing menthols of peppermint, they each offer a different sensory stimulus for the palate and different healing properties for the body. The best way to learn more about these healing culinary herbs is to experiment with them in small quantities.

## Aloe Vera

Aloe Vera is a good source of vitamins A, B1, B2, B3, B6, B12, folate, calcium, zinc, magnesium and potassium.

Excellent for skin health, anti-tumor, anti-inflammatory, antibiotic and analgesic. Aloe supports balanced blood sugar levels, immune function, and alkalizes the body. Aloe is recognized as one of the ten major superfoods and has a 5,000 year history as a medicinal plant. It was known in ancient Egyptian times as the plant of immortality.

## Basil

Excellent source of vitamin K, very good source of iron, calcium and vitamin A, and a good source of manganese, magnesium, potassium, and vitamins B6 and C. The volatile oils and flavonoids in basil have been shown to be anti-microbial and anti-bacterial, even restricting the growth of staphylococcus. Washing produce in a 1% solution of Basil essential oil can eliminate the risk of certain plant born bacterial illnesses. Adding Basil to raw produce drinks and salads can provide anti-bacterial protection.

## Cinnamon

Very good source of manganese and calcium. Cinnamon is anti-inflammatory, anti-fungal, anti-microbial and effective in controlling blood sugar levels. It also binds to bile salts in the digestive tract, helping to remove bile and lower cholesterol. Cinnamon acts on blood platelets to avoid excessive clumping. The scent of cinnamon also increases brain function.

## Ginger

Ginger is an excellent anti-inflammatory due to the compound known as "gingerol" which gives ginger its distinct taste and healing action. Research with arthritis patients has demonstrated marked decrease in swelling and pain in arthritis sufferers using ginger. It has also been proven highly effective against nausea and abdominal discomfort including bloating and gas. Studies have demonstrated it is also very effective against motion sickness and in fact has been proven more effective than Dramamine, the number one over the counter motion sickness product. Additionally, gingerol also seems to be proving out as a significant anti-tumor substance based on research with mice where tumors either failed to form or were significantly smaller in mice treated with gingerol as compared to untreated mice.

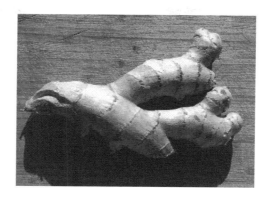

## Mint

Very good source of vitamin A, and a good source of manganese, and vitamin C.

Peppermint is probably most well-known for its ability to soothe an upset stomach. Studies have shown it is effective in soothing IBS and other inflammatory disorders. Anti-inflammatory, anti-bacterial, antioxidant - peppermint also provides relief by supporting open airways and easier breathing in asthma patients. Monoterpene, a substance found in peppermint oil, has been shown to stop the growth of liver, mammary and pancreatic tumors in animal studies.

## Oregano

Excellent source of vitamin K, and a very good source of manganese, iron calcium and vitamin E.

Most well-known for its anti-bacterial action, Oil of Oregano has been sold in health food stores for many years. If you've ever followed a Candida cleanse, you may well recognize it as one of the ingredients in the regimen. Oregano oil is well established as an anti-bacterial and super antioxidant. It has even been found to be more effective than the prescription treatment of Giardia lamblia in a study in Mexico.

## Rosemary

Good source of iron and calcium.

Rosemary is good for your skin and hair and has a long history of stimulating hair growth. It is also known for its stimulation of blood flow to the brain, improving your mental focus and clarity. Rosemary contains many healing substances known to combat headache, muscle aches and fatigue. Historically it has been used as an anti-spasmodic as well as in the treatment of skin ulcers, wounds and eczema. New research is demonstrating it may be helpful in reducing the severity of asthma attacks.

## Thyme

Excellent source of vitamin K, iron and manganese, very good source of calcium.

Thyme has been studied for its antispasmodic properties, as well as its high antioxidant value. Thyme oil has also been shown to be highly antimicrobial, sharing some of the same properties as Rosemary.

## Turmeric

Excellent source of manganese and iron, good source of vitamin B6 and potassium.

Turmeric has now been shown to be not only an important cancer preventive but also anti-tumor, anti-inflammatory and pain relieving. It is quickly becoming the new superstar of the healing plant kingdom. It has been shown to soothe IBS, and to prevent the plaque build-up that causes Alzheimer's disease. It's also been shown to alleviate rheumatoid arthritis and cystic fibrosis. The health benefits of this versatile peppery bright yellow root of the Curcuma Longa plant are now under so much study that its health benefits list just keeps growing. From potentially preventing childhood leukemia to reducing or eliminating symptoms of arthritis, the list just keeps growing. At the same time, turmeric is becoming more readily available in its raw root form, which is excellent for juicing.

Turmeric is definitely an acquired taste, but due to its extreme health benefits, well worth the effort. We have tried it in many different juices and variations and have found the absolute best juice recipe for turmeric is the one to be found at Food Babe's website (http://foodbabe.com), which we are placing here in the book with a link to her site. As an aside, we totally love FoodBabe, and have had a lot of fun exploring her world of food and juicing. Her recipe for a tasty zesty and zippy juice that includes a healthy helping of turmeric is a real achievement. We've mixed lemon, parsley and other juice ingredients in our juices along with the turmeric to help mellow the taste, but only her juice recipe seems to actually transform it into something that doesn't just taste to me like a great juice with turmeric added. I'm not sure what the secret is, or why, but what I do know is, I can drink FoodBabe's Turmeric Cooler anytime and really ENJOY it.

Perhaps it's the romaine, or the cucumber and lemon combination, I don't know. I only know this is a really delicious, light and zesty drink. And it works! Thanks FoodBabe.

http://foodbabe.com/2013/01/29/turmeric-cooler-an-anti-inflammatory-juice/

Ingredients:

2 inch piece of turmeric
1 bunch romaine lettuce
3 carrots
1 cucumber with ends removed
1 lemon with peel removed

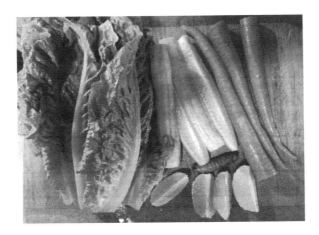

Instructions:

Wash all vegetables thoroughly and place into a large bowl. Juice each vegetable in this order: turmeric, romaine, carrots, lemon, and cucumber. Stir mixture before serving. Clean juicer immediately.

# A Note about the Ratings Used in this Chapter

There are a lot of rating systems out there for foods and nutrients, most provided through FDA, USDA and other governmental sources. However, the work of *The George Mateljan Foundation* for *The World's Healthiest Foods*, has, in our opinion, developed the most comprehensive and accurate ratings system for nutrient density and caloric intake.

Here is how their system works:

Good: Foods rated 'Good' for any nutrient must contain 1.5 times the daily requirement for that nutrient than the percentage of caloric intake they require.

Very Good: Foods rated 'Very Good' must deliver the nutrient value for that nutrient rated very good at 3.5 times the percentage of daily caloric value they require.

Excellent: Foods rated excellent must provide 7.5 times more nutrient value than the caloric intake they require.

In other words, if a serving of the food described uses 10% of the daily caloric value, in order to be rated for the three ratings the nutrient being rated must deliver 15%, 35% or 75% of the daily nutrient requirement for that nutrient in order for the food to be rated as the good, very good or excellent source of that nutrient.

This helps to distinguish the most nutrient dense foods easily and provides a uniform rating system across all foods.

To learn more about the Foundation's rating system, visit their rating system questions and answers page online at:

http://www.whfoods.com/genpage.php?tname=faq&dbid=22#how1

# Care and Maintenance Tips for Your Omega Juicer

## A Few Do's and Don'ts in Juicer Care

- **Do** always disconnect and clean the juicing part of your juicer immediately after every use. If you cannot immediately clean it completely, at least separate all parts and rinse them so no pulp is standing inside the workings of the machine, and then come back and give it a thorough washing later.

- **Do** shut the juicer off in between juicing portions. If you are cutting up large pieces of apples or other produce which will not fit into the juicing chute, shut the juicer off while you chop and then turn it back on when you are ready to start juicing again. This reduces un-necessary wear and overheating of the motor.

- **Do** run the switch backward for a moment if you feel that produce is getting jammed inside the masticator compartment. Sometimes it will seem as if things are a little stuck and not moving forward as you'd like. Just flip the power switch into reverse for a moment and then back to the on/forward position to dislodge any obstructions and continue juicing. You might also juice a carrot or harder fruit or vegetable to help push softer, stickier things through.

- **Do** rinse the juicer's juicing parts over the garbage disposal or compost bin first, before you wash it in the sink, to remove the pulp that would otherwise clog your normal sink's drain. When rinsing the smaller parts of the juicer over the disposal sink, be careful not to drop them down into the large drain opening of the disposal where they could be damaged or broken. (Ask us how we know this one.) Once the parts are all rinsed, wash them in your regular sink with hot soapy water.

- **Do** use the specialized scrubbing brush that resembles a rather large toothbrush that came with your juicer to brush out the mesh portions of the juicing screen and along the ridgelines of the masticator. It is very important to remove all food and pulp from these areas to get a really clean machine and not transfer soap particles, pulp and other debris back to the juicer.

- **Do** rinse all the juicing parts thoroughly with hot water after washing to make sure there is no soap residue left on any part of the machine.

- **Do not** ever wash the motor body of the machine. Wipe it with a slightly moist cloth only. Never allow any liquid to get on the top of the machine where the power switch is, as water could enter the power switch and short it out. One of the wonderful things about the Omega juicer is that it comes with a full 10 year warranty on all parts. This is really almost unheard of in today's world of 'planned obsolescence' products. And they back up that warranty with a friendly, easy to reach customer service department. About a year after we bought our juicer, we managed to break the juicing screen that is used for making the juice. It was really our fault, although we didn't want to admit it - we dropped it down the disposal drain side of the sink and broke it trying to get it back out. But one phone call and not only did Omega send us a replacement, they sent us two! We still have that extra one in the drawer, in case we somehow manage to break the first replacement.

- Your Omega juicer comes with a small plastic bag containing the assortments of extrusion nozzles and caps for use with making frozen desserts, pasta, nut butters and baby foods. There is also a "blank cone" which is the juicing insert for the masticating cylinder with no screens. This allows you to make specialty food preparations without separating the juice out of them.

# Bibliography

There are well over two dozen books in our library on nutrition, health, food and juicing, and to some degree they have all contributed to this book; however, the books which were actual references for fact checking and for the foundational understanding which allowed me to write this book are the two listed here.

## Books

- The Encyclopedia of Healing Foods, 2005, Dr. Michael T. Murray
- The Gerson Therapy: The Proven Nutritional Program for Cancer and Other Illnesses, 2001, Charlotte Gerson and Morton Walker

## Online Sources

- Natural News.com:
  http://www.naturalnews.com/021858_aloe_vera_gel.html
- http://scholar.google.com/scholar?q=aloe+vera+blood&btnG=&hl=en&as_sdt=0%2C38
- Indian Journal of Experimental Biology, Vol. 37, February 1999, pp.124-131
- Pharmacology of rosemary (Rosmarinus officinalis Linn.) and its therapeutic potentials, M R Al-Sereitia, K M Abu-Amerb & P Sena

- Nutritional Profile for Barley Grass (one example): http://www.druworldwide.com/natural_foods/dru_barleygrass_nutritional_info

- Wheatgrass facts and benefits: http://www.mywheatgrass.com/wheatgrass-facts-benefits.shtml

- Worlds Healthiest Foods - In-Depth Nutrition Information, Data and Food Preparation Recommendations: http://www.whfoods.com/foodstoc.php

- Chris Kresser L. Ac: http://chriskresser.com/folate-vs-folic-acid

# Recommended Reading

## Books

- The Encyclopedia of Healing Foods, 2005 , Michael T. Murray
- Complete Book of Juicing: Your Delicious Guide to Youthful Vitality, 1997, Michael T. Murray
- The Gerson Therapy: The Proven Nutritional Program for Cancer and Other Illnesses, 2001, Charlotte Gerson and Morton Walker
- Healing the Gerson Way : Defeating Cancer and Other Chronic Diseases, 2009, Charlotte Gerson
- Gerson Therapy Recipes with Detailed Cooking Instructions, 1991, Charlotte Gerson
- Juicing, Fasting, and Detoxing for Life: Unleash the Healing Power of Fresh Juices and Cleansing Diets, Cherie Calbom, 2008

## Online Sources

- Local Harvest - the nonprofit reference guide for farmers markets, CSA's and fresh local produce:
  http://www.localharvest.org/
- Folate Vs Folic Acid: The Little Known but Important Difference Between Folate and Folic Acid:
  http://chriskresser.com/folate-vs-folic-acid

- The Juice Nut - this is a fun site with lots of juice recipes and some good advice from a fellow who is, well, nuts about juicing - http://www.thejuicenut.com/
- Worlds Healthiest Foods – In-Depth Nutrition Information, Data and Food Preparation Recommendations: http://www.whfoods.com/foodstoc.php (On the information page for each food listed there is a Nutritional Profile section which links to a complete in-depth nutritional analysis of the food item.) Extensive research data and complete references make this perhaps the most useful online resource for healthy eating. Their data is derived from Food Processor for Windows, Version 7.60, by ESHA Research in Salem, Oregon, USA.

29336990R00089

Made in the USA
Lexington, KY
22 January 2014